INTERMITTENT FASTING

Intermittent Fasting for Women Over 50

All You need to Know (and Avoid) to Achieve Permanent Weight Loss, Detox Your Body and Make your Friends Jealous!

By Victoria Robson

TABLE OF CONTENTS

INTRODUCTION

Diet fads abound around the world. Diet pills were popular in the 1990s. In the early 2000s, if you didn't have a juicer, you were losing out on some of life's most crucial health-promoting ingredients. We have been gifted green tea pads that reduce tummy size, and if you're not eating like a Neanderthal, you're already at a disadvantage. As a general rule, I am extremely dubious of all fads. Suppose anything is being hailed as innovative and game-changing in the field of weight reduction. In that case, chances are it is merely marketing lingo to promote whatever is now popular in the industry. When it comes to diet trends, intermittent fasting is one that I am eager to discuss with you since it is a trend that I believe will last for a long time.

When it comes to losing weight, women over 50 often have difficulties. A variety of factors can cause this. The primary cause of this condition is frequently a sluggish metabolism. The greater the amount of lean muscle mass you have, the faster your metabolism. However, as we grow older, we lose lean muscle mass and become less physically active than we were previously. As a result, what happened? It's hard to lose stubborn body fat that just won't budge.

Intermittent fasting has become popular in recent years due to its range of health benefits and not restricting your food choices. According to research, fasting can help you lose weight, enhance your mental health, and might help you avoid certain malignancies. It can also help prevent certain muscle, nerve, and joint diseases in women over the age of 50.

Women over the age of 50 who practice intermittent fasting can experience weight loss and reduce the risk of acquiring age-related ailments. According to a new study conducted by Baylor College of Medicine, intermittent fasting can help to reduce blood pressure levels. According to the findings of the study, fasting can reduce blood pressure via altering the gut flora.

Of course, many women over the age of 50 are concerned about losing weight and trying to improve their health. It is more difficult to lose weight after the age of 50 for various reasons, including decreased metabolic rate, achy joints, decreased muscle mass, and even sleep troubles. Meanwhile, lowering weight – particularly hazardous belly fat – can significantly lower your chance of developing major health problems such as diabetes, heart disease, and cancer.

Of course, as you become older, your chances of having a variety of ailments grow. In certain situations, intermittent fasting for women over 50 can act as a genuine fountain of youth when it comes to weight loss and reducing the risk of acquiring age-related ailments such as heart disease and diabetes.

Chapter 1: HISTORY OF INTERMITTENT FASTING

Fasting is not a new notion. Humans have fasted for various reasons, including nighttime periods, religious reasons, and food scarcity. Fasting is said to be one of the oldest therapeutic practices in the world. Hippocrates of Cos, a Greek philosopher, advocated fasting. Other Greek philosophers, such as Plato and Aristotle, were major supporters of fasting. Fasting was thought to be a universal tendency for various ailments by the ancient Greeks. They also believed that it enhanced cognitive ability. Consider a day when your tummy was overflowing with food. Did you feel intellectually alert and energized afterward, or were you tired and sleepy?

Fasting is used to wash or purify the soul in various faiths (including Islam, Christianity, and Buddhism). However, it effectively translates into the identical advantages that the Greek researchers have approved.

Modern intermittent fasting is all about progressively adopting fasting into your daily diet. It entails eating wisely most of the time and then going without food for an extended time now and then. You can also have cheat days once a week, where you can overeat a restricted quantity of food.

Reduce the Eating Window Length

According to research, the timing of intermittent fasting is important. Our eating window typically begins with breakfast at 7:00 a.m. and ends at 8:00 p.m. with our last meal/snack. The concept behind intermittent fasting is to simply minimize that eating window, not necessarily eating less every time but more often. Most dieticians believe that including an 8-hour eating window or fasting for sixteen hours can help a person perceive the advantages of IF. This implies that you can eat your lunch at noon and your final snack at 8:00 p.m., and that's it for IF.

It must now make you consider all the bad health consequences of missing breakfast. Breakfast has long been regarded as the essential meal of the day. That is correct. Clean diet is required for IF to be effective. Even if your eating window opens, you will no longer be overeating once your body has been acclimated to it.

The nicest part about IF is that it is completely free. All you have to do now is adjust to a new eating method. There's no need to spend money on a guide, equipment, or supplements. If you're thinking about taking supplements, Zanesville Medical Center has extensive health-boosting formulations and supplements assessments.

Don't Deny, but Delay

The nicest part about IF is that you are not depriving yourself of food; rather, you are delaying it. When your eating window opens, you can have a piece of pizza (not the entire box) or a scoop of ice cream. While you must remain sensible even throughout your eating window, there are no exceptions, which is a thrilling prospect. Fasting can appear challenging on paper, but it is far simpler to practice than diets.

Your expenditure will also be reduced as a result of IF. When you reduce your eating habits to one or two meals per day, you begin to save for additional costs such as a down payment on a new automobile, a weekend getaway to the countryside, or updating the interior of your house.

Where Do I Begin?

When it comes to IF, there are two schools of thinking. One method asks for a 5:2 diet, in which you eat normally for 5 days and then fast for 2 days. The alternative method is the 16:8 structure, which we discussed before. The most crucial component of IF is to keep it clean, not only quick. The goal is to deny your body any sweets, carbohydrates, or fats that might cause insulin production. There are no extra fats or sweets allowed in your tea, water, or coffee. It's difficult at first, but the end product is well worth it.

If you've tried other diets and they haven't worked for you, I recommend trying IF to enhance your general health. It's worth a go because it's free and can save you money.

THE SCIENCE BEHIND INTERMITTENT FASTING

Intermittent fasting has been regarded as the answer to weight loss, and you've heard the buzz.

But what is the truth?

According to senior researcher Satchin Panda, while there is legitimate scientific evidence for intermittent fasting's advantages, it is neither a quick nor a definite remedy. Panda, a professor of circadian biology at the Salk Institute for Biological Studies in La Jolla, California, has dedicated his career researching the human body's complicated biochemical processes. Intermittent fasting appears to boost human health in various ways, including weight loss, according to his study in mice and humans.

Before we go into the research, let's be clear: there is no one-size-fits-all approach to intermittent fasting. If you Google it, you'll find many alternatives, each with its own set of supporters. The 5: 2 diet includes eating extremely few calories (about 500-600) on two days of the week, then eating normally for five days. Alternate-day fasting is another option, which involves eating normally one day and then eating nothing or perhaps 500 calories.

All intermittent fasting strategies work on the same principle: your body will turn to stored fat for energy when your calorie intake is reduced. However, intermittent fasting differs from calorie restriction. It could be simpler for people to restrict calories for short periods rather than the days, weeks, and months required by traditional diets. Plus, the form of intermittent fasting Panda investigated might provide extra benefits.

Panda has been focusing on a type of intermittent fasting called time-restricted feeding. A person consumes all of their calories for the day during an 8-to-12-hour span. Let's pretend you start your day with a cup of coffee at 7 a.m. and end it with popcorn and a drink at 11 p.m. You could move to eating breakfast at 8 a.m., including coffee, and finishing your supper by 6 p.m. if you practice time-restricted eating. You'll be eating all of your meals within a 10-hour timeframe, and you'll be skipping desserts, nighttime snacks, and alcohol calories. But it isn't the end of the narrative.

Time-restricted eating appears to be beneficial to the body more than just calorie reduction. Panda and colleagues' mouse research from 2012 was the first to demonstrate this. They took two genetically identical sets of mice and fed them the same diet — a lab-mice version of the standard American diet high in fat and simple sugar and low in protein.

While both groups were given an identical amount of food, one group had access to it for 24 hours while the other only had access for 8 hours. Mice are nocturnal creatures that sleep during the day and feed at night. When one set of mice was given access to food 24 hours a day, they began consuming part of it during the day, when they should have been sleeping.

The mice who could feed exhibited evidence of insulin resistance and liver damage after 18 weeks. These circumstances did not exist in the mice who ate within an 8-hour interval. They also weighed 28% less than mice that had access to food 24 hours a day, although both groups of mice consumed the same number of calories each day. Panda says, "It was kind of earth-shattering." He and other academics believed that weight gain was governed by the overall quantity of calories consumed rather than when they were consumed.

The experiment was repeated with three additional groups of mice, and the findings were the same. The results were consistent across different types of food and feeding periods of up to 15 hours, albeit the shorter the window, the less weight the mice acquired. When the time-restricted mice were given free rein for two days a week, or what Panda refers to as "taking the weekend off," they acquired less weight than mice permitted to eat 24 hours a day.

Panda's team then tried another way: they swapped mice who gained weight due to unlimited feeding and time-restricted eating. Despite ingesting the same number of calories, these mice dropped weight and kept it off for the duration of the research, which was 12 weeks. They also lowered insulin resistance, which is known to be connected to fat, but experts are still puzzled by the relationship. Of course, the human body is more sophisticated than a mouse's, but these trials were the first hint of how crucial timing might be for how our bodies utilize food, according to Panda.

According to experts, many of the human body's activities have been linked to our circadian rhythms in recent years. Most of us are aware that obtaining sunshine first thing in the morning is good for our mood and sleep and that being exposed to light after 9 p.m. via our mobile phones or computers can disrupt our night's sleep. "Similarly, the correct food at the right time can nourish us, whereas the wrong food at the wrong moment might be junk food," Panda explains. It is stored as fat instead of being used as fuel, which makes sense when considering the foundations of human metabolism.

Time-restricted eating allows our bodies to burn fat for longer periods. Our bodies use carbs for energy when we eat, and if we don't use them immediately, they are stored as glycogen in the liver or turned into fat. Our bodies run on glucose from the carbs we've just eaten for a few hours after we've done eating for the day before dipping into stored carbohydrates, or glycogen, in the liver. Our bodies' glycogen stores persist for several hours before running out around eight hours after we stop eating, at which point our bodies start to draw into their fat reserves.

We spend more time in this fat-burning stage of our metabolism when we decrease our eating window and increase our fasting window. However, as soon as we consume food again — even if it's only a cup of coffee with a little sugar and milk — we revert to the other mode, burning carbs and storing glycogen and fat. So, if you complete your evening snack at 10 p.m., your body will run out of glycogen and begin burning fat at 6 a.m. If you modify your breakfast time from 6 a.m. to 9 a.m., you've given your body three more hours to burn fat for fuel.

Panda tested his time-restricted eating trials on people and discovered that they were as promising. In 2015, he and his colleagues attempted to put a small sample of people on a 16-week time-restricted eating schedule. Surprisingly, the researchers provided these folks with no nutrition guidance or instructions. Instead, the participants were instructed to eat just during a 10- to 12-hour timeframe. They snapped photographs of their meal and sent them to the researchers while they ate. The patients lost a little amount of weight — an average of slightly over 8 pounds apiece — after 16 weeks.

According to Panda, they reported better sleep, greater energy in the mornings, and less hunger at bedtime, implying that time-restricted eating "really has a systemic influence throughout the body." While the sample size was much too small to draw clear results, the researchers were encouraged that the modest intervention appeared to be straightforward for patients to execute and maintain.

Time-restricted eating has been demonstrated to reduce the risk of diabetes. Panda and his team discovered that after one week of restricting their meals to a nine-hour window, 15 men at risk for type-2 diabetes had a smaller jump in blood glucose following a test meal, indicating greater insulin sensitivity. It could also aid in the reduction of cholesterol. Panda and colleagues time-restricted the eating of 19 patients, most of whom were taking medication to decrease cholesterol, blood pressure, or diabetes. They reduced their overall cholesterol by roughly 11% on average after 12 weeks of eating within a 10-hour timeframe. Panda also checked in a year later and discovered that around 34% of the individuals were still eating willingly in an 8-11 hour timeframe. "It was great that they could self-sustain for such a long time," Panda adds. This is good news because, according to some estimates, 13 to 12 percent of dieters gain back more weight than they lost.

According to Panda, here's how you can practice time-restricted eating. While some intermittent fasting strategies enable people to drink as much coffee and tea as they like during the day, he recommends that you just drink water during your fasting window. This means no coffee, tea, or herbal tea, all of which can alter blood chemistry and are thus prohibited during medical blood testing.

Panda suggests drinking simple hot water after waking up; it can have a similar relaxing effect as coffee. However, if you need to be awake in the morning, he says it's fine to enjoy a cup of black coffee — just avoid adding creamer, sugar, honey, or other sweets. "Just one teaspoon of sugar is enough to increase our blood sugar," he claims, causing your body to switch from fat-burning to carb-burning mode.

Panda suggests that you delay eating breakfast until you've been up for hours. The hormone cortisol surges around 45 minutes after waking up, and excessive cortisol levels can impair glucose management. Furthermore, the hormone melatonin, which prepares our bodies for sleep, only lasts two hours after we wake up. This implies that your pancreas, which creates the insulin required to utilize carbs in food, wakes up for the first two hours. Then, two to three hours before bedtime, attempt to finish your last meal since this is when melatonin begins to prepare the body, especially your pancreas, for sleep.

While intermittent fasting, particularly time-restricted eating, has intriguing potential, it is still early. Other study organizations have backed up some of Panda's findings since he began his studies. According to research published in Cell Metabolism in July, people on a time-restricted eating regimen lowered their calorie intake despite not being asked to and dropped a little weight.

More study into time-restricted eating is required. There haven't been any human subjects studies that have lasted more than a few months thus far. According to researchers, fasting's effects on the human body must also be understood.

The gut microbiome, for example, has been found to shift in mice who restrict their feeding to an eight-to-nine-hour window, causing them to process nutrients differently and absorb less sugar and fat. Is this something that humans can do? That will have to wait and see. Panda isn't the only one looking into the long-term implications of time-restricted eating; other academics are starting to look into whether intermittent fasting might protect the brain from neurodegenerative illnesses.

Intermittent fasting isn't a magic weight-loss solution. According to several studies, those who follow the 5:2 diet or alternate-day fasting can automatically eat more before and after their fasting days and lower their activity on fasting days, offsetting the calorie-cutting effects. Panda claims that in his research on time-restricted eating, he's observed some people gain weight after taking the concept of eating anything they wanted inside a window to its logical conclusion, bingeing on items they normally avoid. In addition, unlike mice, the human body seems to have mechanisms for slowing metabolism to burn fewer calories as you consume fewer. Finally, whether or not intermittent fasting is advantageous to persons who aren't attempting to reduce weight is unknown. Persons who suffer from binge-eating disorder or anorexia could be at risk; it's easy to understand how adopting intermittent fasting might foster these destructive behaviors.

Time-restricted eating provides several advantages over other weight loss methods: It's simple. Diets are generally the privilege of those who can afford them since many individuals don't have the time or means to count calories — plan their meals, buy particular foods, track their calories. Anyone who can measure time and limit eating and drinking to specified intervals can practice time-restricted eating.

Panda and his colleagues are currently recruiting 120 people to participate in time-restricted eating research. They are also looking at whether firefighters' health can be improved by eating for 10 hours. Due to the frequent disturbance of their circadian rhythms, firefighters and other shift workers are more susceptible to illness.

People who wish to lose weight have focused on adjusting their everyday diets for a long time. Time-restricted eating can broaden the range of variables within our control. Panda, who follows a 10-hour eating window, adds, "When it comes to health, we have a variety of possibilities." "Now, we can include food time in the menu."

Intermittent fasting (IF), for example, is an efficient way to keep and improve a healthy lifestyle. Fasting can be done for various reasons, including weight loss, detoxification, and religious reasons. There has been a significant quantity of scientific studies supporting the health advantages of fasting. Although it has mostly been tested on animals, the results are encouraging. Fasting lowers oxidative stress, improves memory, retains learning, and improves disease biomarkers.

Chapter 2: INTERMITTENT FASTING

Intermittent fasting is a form of eating plan in which you alternate between fasting and normal meals. Intermittent fasting has been shown in studies to help individuals lose weight and prevent — or even reverse — illness. How do you go about achieving that? Is it also safe?

While many diets focus on what to eat, intermittent fasting focuses on when to eat.

When you fast intermittently, you only eat at particular periods of the day. Fat reduction may be aided by fasting for a predetermined number of hours each day or eating just one meal a couple of times each week. Scientific evidence also shows that there are certain health advantages.

For the last 25 years, Mark Mattson, a neurologist at Johns Hopkins University, has studied intermittent fasting. He claims that our bodies have grown to be able to survive without food for several hours, days, or even weeks. Before humans discovered how to farm, they were hunters and gatherers who adapted to survive and thrive without eating for lengthy periods. They had to: Hunting wildlife and gathering berries and nuts took time and effort.

Maintaining a healthy weight was easy, even 50 years ago. "There were no computers, and TV programs switched off at 11 p.m.; people stopped eating because they went to bed," explains Christie Williams, M.S., R.D.N., a Johns Hopkins nutritionist. The portions were somewhat smaller. "More people went outdoors to work and play, getting more exercise."

Television, the internet, and other types of entertainment are now accessible 24 hours a day, 7 day of the week. We stay up longer to watch our favorite programs, play video games, and converse online. We sit and nibble for the whole day — and most of the night."

Eating too many calories and exercising too little can aggravate obesity, heart disease, type 2 diabetes, and other ailments. In scientific studies, intermittent fasting has been proven to aid in the reversal of these patterns.

HOW DOES IT WORK?

Intermittent fasting can be accomplished in a various ways, but they all center on establishing regular eating and fasting schedules. You could, for example, only eat for eight hours a day and fast the rest of the time. You might also limit yourself to one meal each day, two times per week. You can pick from a range of intermittent fasting regimens.

According to Mattson, the body's sugar reserves are exhausted over a period without food, and it starts to burn fat. He refers to this as "metabolic switching."

"Because most Americans eat constantly throughout their waking hours," Mattson argues, "intermittent fasting is in sharp contrast to their typical eating regimen." "If someone eats three meals a day, including snacks, and does not exercise, they are burning calories but not removing fat reserves every time they eat."

Intermittent fasting works by extending the period between when your body burns the calories from your last meal and when it begins to burn fat.

HOW INTERMITTENT FASTING HELPS IN WEIGHT LOSS

Losing weight can be done in various ways. Intermittent fasting has become more fashionable in recent years.

Intermittent fasting is usually associated with weight reduction. Fasting for short periods of time consumes less calories, resulting in weight reduction over time.

However, intermittent fasting can help reduce risk factors for diabetes and cardiovascular disease by reducing cholesterol and blood sugar levels.

Choosing an Intermittent Fasting Plan

IF can be done in various ways. Among the most popular are:

- the 16:8 system

- the 5:2 eating plan

- Warrior's Diet

- Stop eating and start eating again

- Alternate day fasting (ADF)

All of the strategies can be beneficial, but figuring out which one works best for you is a personal choice.

Here's a review of each strategy's advantages and disadvantages to help you determine which is best for you.

THE 16/8 METHOD

The 16/8 intermittent fasting approach is one of the most popular weight reduction fasting strategies. The diet restricts food and calorie-containing beverages to an 8-hour window each day. It requires fasting for the remaining 16 hours of the day.

The 16/8 approach is more flexible and is based on a time-restricted feeding (TRF) concept, while other diets can have rigorous limitations and regulations.

You can consume calories over any 8-hour period.

Some people avoid eating after 5 p.m. and adhere to a 9 a.m. to 5 p.m. schedule, while others skip breakfast and fast from 12 p.m. to 8 p.m.

Limiting the amount of hours you can eat each day will help you lose weight and lower your blood pressure.

According to studies, time-restricted meal patterns, such as the 16/8 method, can help people avoid hypertension and eat less, resulting in weight reduction.

According to a 2016 study, the 16/8 strategy helped male participants shed fat while maintaining muscle mass, When combined with weight exercise.

A more recent research found that the 16/8 technique had no effect on muscle or strength gains in women who completed resistance training.

While the 16/8 approach can easily be integrated into any lifestyle, some individuals find going 16 hours without eating challenging.

Furthermore, eating too many junk food OR snacks during your 8-hour fasting window can negate the 16/8 intermittent fasting benefits. Consume a well-balanced diet rich in fruits, whole grains, vegetables, healthy fats, and protein to gain the maximum health benefits from this diet.

THE 5:2 METHOD

The 5:2 diet is a simple intermittent fasting plan.

You eat five days a week without counting calories. Then, you reduce your calorie intake to one-quarter of your daily needs on the other two days of the week.

For someone who eats 2,000 calories daily, this would entail cutting their calorie consumption to 500 calories two days per week.

According to a 2018 study, the 5:2 diet is equally as efficient for weight reduction and blood glucose management in people with type 2 diabetes as daily calorie restriction.

Another study revealed that the 5:2 diet was equally efficient for weight reduction and preventing metabolic disorders, including diabetes, heart disease, and as continuous calorie restriction.

The 5:2 diet allows you to choose which days you fast, and there are no restrictions on what or when you eat on full-calorie days.

It's worth noting that eating "normally" on full-calorie days does not imply that you could eat everything you want.

Even if it is only for two days a week, limiting oneself to 500 calories a day is difficult. Furthermore, eating too few calories can cause you to become faint or unwell.

The 5:2 diet could be useful for some people, but it is not for everyone. Consult doctor to find out whether the 5:2 diet is right for you.

EAT, STOP, EAT

Brad Pilon, author of "Eat Stop Eat," advocated for a novel intermittent fasting strategy called "Eat Stop Eat."

This approach of intermittent fasting comprises selecting on one or two non-consecutive days each week when you will fast for 24 hours. The remainder of the week is yours to eat as much as you like, but it's ideal to eat a well-balanced diet and avoid overindulging.

The belief that consuming fewer calories would result in weight reduction justifies a weekly 24-hour fast.

Fasting for up to 24 hours might cause a metabolic shift, leading your body to use fat as an energy source rather than glucose.

However, abstaining from meals for 24 hours takes a lot of discipline and might lead to bingeing and overeating later. It might also result in disturbed eating habits.

More study is needed to establish the Eat Stop Eat diet's possible health advantages and weight reduction qualities.

Consult your doctor before you attempt Eat Stop Eat to determine whether it's a good weight-loss plan.

ALTERNATE-DAY FASTING

Alternate-day fasting is a basic, easy-to-follow IF diet. On this diet, you fast every other day but eat anything you want on the non-fasting days.

Some variations of this diet use a "modified" fasting strategy, in which fasting days are accompanied with a 500-calorie meal. Other variations, on the other hand, totally exclude calories on fasting days.

People who fast on alternate days have been found to lose weight.

Alternate-day fasting was shown to be as effective for weight reduction as daily calorie restriction in a randomized pilot study of obese persons.

Another study found that after four weeks of alternating between 36 hours of fasting and 12 hours of unrestricted eating, people consumed 35% less calories and lost an average of 7.7 pounds (3.5 kg).

If you're serious about losing weight, incorporating an exercise program into your everyday routine will help you lose weight.

Combining alternate-day fasting with endurance exercise, according to study, can result in weight reduction that is twice as effective as just fasting.

Fasting for a entire day every other day might be difficult, particularly if you're new to it. It's easy to overindulge on non-fasting days.

If you're new to intermittent fasting, start with a modified fasting regimen to ease into alternate-day fasting.

It is ideal for maintaining a balanced diet, containing high protein meals and low-calorie veggies to help you feel full, whether you start with a full fast or a modified fasting plan.

THE WARRIOR DIET

The Warrior Diet is an IF strategy based on the feeding practices of ancient warriors.

Ori Hofmekler created the Warrior Diet in 2001, which is more severe than the 16:8 approach but less so than the Eat Fast Eat method.

It requires eating very little for 20 hours during the day and then eating as much as you like for a 4-hour window at night.During the 20-hour fast, the Warrior Diet advises dieters to take tiny amounts of dairy products, hard-boiled eggs, raw fruits, vegetables, and non-calorie drinks.

People can eat anything they want during a 4-hour window after a 20-hour fast, although unprocessed, nutritious, and organic meals are encouraged.

While no study has been done on the Warrior Diet specifically, human studies have shown that time-restricted meal cycles can help people lose weight.

Other health advantages of time-restricted eating cycles are unknown. In rodents, time-restricted feeding cycles have been shown to prevent diabetes, decrease tumor growth, delay aging, and extend longevity.

More study on the Warrior Diet is needed to comprehend its weight-loss advantages properly.

The Warrior Diet could be tough to stick to since it limits calorie intake to only 4 hours each day. Overeating late at night is a common problem.

The Warrior Diet has been linked to eating disorders. Whether you're up for the task, see your doctor determine if it is appropriate for you.

Consult your doctor before initiating intermittent fasting. The actual process is simple once you have his or her consent. You might opt for a daily plan that restricts daily meals to a six- to eight-hour window. For instance, you could attempt 16/8 fasting, which involves eating for eight hours and fasting for sixteen. Williams supports the daily routine, claiming that most individuals find it simple to stay in this pattern over time.

Another method is to eat five times a week, which is known as the 5:2 technique. On the following two days, you only consume one 500–600 calorie meal. Assume you decide to eat normally every day of the week except Mondays and Thursdays, when you will have just one meal.

Fasting for extended periods of time, such as 24 hours, 36 hours, 48 hours, or 72 hours, is not always healthy and can be dangerous. Going too long without eating could cause your body to begin accumulating fat due to the lack of food.

According to Mattson's studies, it takes 2-4 weeks for the body to adjust to intermittent fasting. While getting adjusted to the new pattern, you can feel hungry or irritable. However, he notes that research subjects which make it through the adjustment stage are more likely to continue with the diet because they feel better.

What effect does IF have on your hormones?

Although intermittent fasting might help you lose weight, it can also have a negative impact on your hormones. This is because body fat is the body's means of storing energy (calories).

When you don't eat, your body goes through a series of adjustments to make its stored energy more available.

Variations in nervous system activity and significant changes in the levels of various important hormones are examples.

When you fast, your metabolism alters in two ways:

• **Insulin:** When you eat, your insulin levels rise, and when you fast, your insulin levels plummet. Insulin levels that are lower aid fat burning.

• **Norepinephrine (noradrenaline):** Norepinephrine is a neurotransmitter that causes fat cells to break down body fat into free fatty acids that can be burnt for energy.

Interestingly, short-term fasting can improve fat burning, contrary to what some proponents of eating 5–6 meals each day suggest.

Alternate-day fasting trials of 3–12 weeks and whole-day fasting trials of 12–24 weeks have been shown to reduce body weight and body fat.

Still, additional study into the long-term implications of intermittent fasting is needed.

Human growth hormone (HGH) is another hormone that changes during a fast, with levels rising to five-fold.

HGH was previously thought to aid fat burning, but new study suggests this could tell the brain to preserve energy, making weight loss more difficult.

HGH can enhance hunger and decrease energy metabolism by stimulating a limited population of agouti-related protein (AgRP) neurons.

Chapter 3: INTERMITTENT FASTING FOR WOMEN OVER 50

One of the main reasons for women over 50 to pursue intermittent fasting is to get greater energy. Many women report a small weight increase and worse sleep quality as they approach menopause. Both of these things might make you sleepy and sluggish. However, you can retrain your body to feel better by modifying when and what you consume.

Both premenopausal and postmenopausal women have benefited from intermittent fasting.

If you are trying to lose weight, IF can help you consume the things you desire when you want the most at night. This means you won't feel starved when watching your favorite shows on TV while everyone else is nibbling.

7 Tips for Women Over 50 Who Want to Fast

Women should consider these pointers over 50 who wants to develop a long-term IF practice.

1: Begin slowly.

Start with a basic overnight fast if you're new to intermittent fasting. To put it another way, go from supper to breakfast without eating anything.

A 12-hour overnight fast requires just 4 hours of wakeful fasting when counting sleep. You can go to lengthier fasts once you've become acclimated to overnight fasting.

2: Consume sufficient calories

Most intermittent fasting studies enable participants to eat as much as they like during feeding windows. Despite this permissive policy, the majority of individuals consume fewer calories overall.

Excessive calorie restriction is unhealthy. Maintain a small caloric deficit of roughly 10% by tracking your meals with the Carb Manager app to avoid exhaustion, sleep difficulties, and other calorie restriction side effects.

3: Make protein a top priority

Inadequate protein consumption hastens the loss of muscle mass as people become older. Sarcopenia (also known as sarcopenia) is a leading source of morbidity in the elderly.

The more you fast, the more difficult it becomes to reach your daily protein goal of 100 grams. (Aiming for 100 grams is a healthy goal for muscle upkeep.) Carb Manager can help you keep track of your protein consumption.

4: Work on your resistance.

All types of exercise can help with IF, but strength training is particularly beneficial. Why? Because strength training helps you keep the lean mass (muscle) that you'd lose if you fast.

As we become older, muscle keeps us functional. And the older we become, the more difficult it is to keep up. By strength training and consuming adequate protein, you can stop this process.

5: Make sure you're getting adequate electrolytes

You lose electrolytes like salt and potassium faster when you fast. Electrolytes must be supplied to avoid headaches, exhaustion, and cramping caused by electrolyte deficit.

Salting your meal, eating electrolyte-rich vegetables like spinach, and maybe taking an electrolyte supplement are all examples of this.

6: Think about going on a Keto diet.

For women over 50, keto and intermittent fasting can be beneficial. Both diets can aid in the reduction of insulin, the promotion of ketosis, and the stimulation of fat loss.

Yes, the Keto diet has been demonstrated to aid weight loss in postmenopausal women.

7: Consume nutrient-dense foods

You must make the most of them because you have fewer opportunities to nourish your body with nutrition while you practice IF.

Fish, Meat, eggs, offal, vegetables, fruits, and healthy fats are examples of nutrient-dense diets. Skip the refined foods and shop the periphery of the supermarket instead.

Chapter 4: INTERMITTENT FASTING BENEFITS

Intermittent fasting can be done in a various ways, including the 16/8 and 5:2 techniques.

It has been proved in several studies to have significant health and cognitive benefits.

Here are eleven health benefits of intermittent fasting that have been scientifically proven.

1. Changes the way hormones, cells, and genes work.

When you don't eat for a long period of time, your body undergoes many changes.

For instance, your body adjusts hormone levels to make stored body fat more accessible while simultaneously launching important cell repair processes.

The following are some of the physiological changes that occur while you fast:

• Insulin concentrations

Insulin levels decrease significantly, allowing fat to be burned more efficiently.

• HGH (human growth hormone) levels

Human growth hormone levels in the blood might skyrocket. Higher amounts of this hormone help with fat burning and muscle building, among other things.

• Cellular regrowth

The body induces important cellular repair actions, such as the removal of waste material from cells.

• Expression of genes

Several genes and substances connected to longevity and disease resistance have been altered in a positive way.

Many of the benefits of intermittent fasting are connected to changes in hormones, gene expression, and cell function.

2. Can help with weight loss and visceral fat reduction.

Many individuals who try intermittent fasting do it in order to lose weight.

In general, intermittent fasting causes you to consume fewer meals.

Unless you compensate by eating much more at other meals, you will consume less calories.

Intermittent fasting also aids weight loss by improving hormone function.

Lower insulin levels, greater HGH levels, and enhanced norepinephrine (noradrenaline) levels help the body burn down fat and utilize it for energy.

As a result, fasting for a brief period increases your metabolic rate, helping you to burn more calories.

In other words, IF works on both sides of the calorie equation. It increases your metabolic rate (calories burned) while lowering the amount of food you eat (reduces calories).

According to a 2014 assessment of the scientific literature, intermittent fasting can result in 3–8% weight loss over 3–24 weeks. This is a massive sum.

Over 6–24 weeks, the research participants lost 4–7% of their waist circumference, indicating that they eliminated visceral fat. The disease-causing fat located in the abdominal cavity is known as visceral fat.

Intermittent fasting-induced less muscle loss than constant calorie restriction, according to a 2011 study.

In 2020, a randomized study looked at individuals who used the 16/8 approach. On this diet, you fast for 16 hours a day and eat within an 8-hour window.

When compared to eating three meals a day, fasting did not result in significant weight loss. After examining a sub - set of the subjects, the researchers discovered that those who fasted lost a significant percentage of their lean mass. This also included lean muscle.

There is a need for more research into the effects of fasting on muscle loss. Intermittent fasting can be a highly effective weight-loss strategy in general.

3. Reduces insulin resistance, which lowers your risk of type 2 diabetes.

In recent decades, type 2 diabetes has become a highly prevalent diagnosis. Its most notable feature is high blood sugar levels in the setting of insulin resistance. Anything that protects against type 2 diabetes and lowers insulin resistance should help lower blood sugar levels.

Intermittent fasting has been shown to have considerable benefits in terms of insulin resistance and blood sugar decrease.

In human studies on IF, fasting blood sugar levels in people with prediabetes were reduced by 3–6% over 8–12 weeks. Insulin levels in the fasting state have been reduced by 20–31%.

According to research, intermittent fasting enhanced survival rates and protected against diabetic retinopathy in mice with diabetes. Diabetic retinopathy is a potentially blinding consequence of diabetes.

This means that intermittent fasting could be extremely beneficial to persons at risk of acquiring type 2 diabetes.

There could, however, be some distinctions between the sexes. In a 2005 study of women, blood sugar control deteriorated following a 22-day intermittent fasting program.

4. Can help the body minimize oxidative stress and inflammation.

Oxidative stress is one of the factors that contribute to aging and many chronic disorders.

It involves unstable chemicals known as free radicals. Free radicals can damage other essential molecules like protein and DNA.

Intermittent fasting has been shown to improve oxidative stress resistance in the body.

Studies have also shown intermittent fasting to help reduce inflammation, which is another major cause of many illnesses.

5. It could be good for your heart.

Heart disease is presently the leading cause of death worldwide.

A number of health indicators (sometimes known as "risk factors") have been linked to a higher or lower risk of heart disease.

Short-term fasting has been shown to help with a number of risk factors, including:

- blood glucose levels

- blood pressure levels

- triglycerides in the blood

- cholesterol levels, both total and LDL (bad) cholesterol

- indicators of inflammation

Much of this, however, is based on animal research. Before any suggestions can be made, additional research into the impact of fasting on heart health in humans is required.

6. Induces a wide range of cellular healing mechanisms.

When we fast, our bodies' cells initiate a process known as autophagy, which is a cellular "waste elimination."

Broken and malfunctioning proteins that accumulate inside cells over time are broken down and metabolized by the cells.

Autophagy has been related to a lower risk of cancer and neurological diseases such as Alzheimer's disease.

7. May aid in the prevention of cancer

Cancer is defined by uncontrolled cell proliferation.

Fasting has been found to offer a number of metabolic benefits, including a lower risk of cancer.

According to promising findings from animal research, IF or diets that imitate fasting can help prevent cancer. Human research has yielded comparable results, albeit additional research is needed.

According to some data, fasting can potentially minimize the negative effects of chemotherapy in people.

ADVANTAGES AND DISADVANTAGES OF INTERMITTENT FASTING

Intermittent fasting (IF) has been used to treat various ailments for ages. There are many types of IF, ranging from plans that exclude meals on specific days to protocols that restrict eating only at specific times of the day.

Even persons who are currently healthy can benefit from these eating habits by achieving and maintaining a healthy weight. The study of the benefits and drawbacks of intermittent fasting is still underway. Long-term research is needed to determine whether this eating regimen produces long-term advantages.

ADVANTAGES

• Simple to Follow

Many dietary plans emphasize consuming some foods while restricting or avoiding others. Learning the exact principles of an eating style might take a significant amount of time. The DASH diet, for example, is the subject of whole books, as are Mediterranean-style meal plans.

You just eat according to the time of day or week on an eating plan that combines intermittent fasting. All you need to know when to eat is a watch or a calendar once you've decided which intermittent fasting strategy is ideal for you.

Why Calorie Counting Isn't Necessary

Some people attempting to lose or maintain a healthy weight would rather not track calories. Measuring portion sizes and calculating daily counts can be time-consuming, whether manually or with a smartphone app.

People are more likely to stick to regimens when pre-measured calorie-controlled items are available, according to a 2011 research.

Jenny Craig and other commercial diets charge a fee for these services. However, many individuals do not have the financial means to pay for such programs, especially in the long run.

Intermittent fasting is a simple option that requires little to no calorie counting. In most cases, calorie restriction (and hence weight reduction) happens due to food being removed or severely restricted on specific days or at certain times of the day.

• There are no Macronutrient Restrictions

Some popular diet programs severely limit certain macronutrients. Many people, for example, follow a low-carb diet to improve their health or lose weight. Others eat a low-fat diet for medical reasons or to lose weight.

These programs demand the client to adopt a new eating pattern, typically substituting new and perhaps unfamiliar items for old favorites. This could need learning new culinary techniques and learning to shop and equip the kitchen in a new way.

Intermittent fasting does not necessitate any of these abilities. No macronutrient range should be targeted, and no macronutrient should be limited or disallowed.

• Unrestricted Consumption

Anyone who has ever tried a new diet understands how much you desire stuff you aren't supposed to consume. An increase in the desire to eat, according to a 2017 study, is a primary driver of failed weight loss attempts.

However, on an intermittent fasting schedule, this issue is much reduced. Food restriction happens just during specific hours of the day, and you can eat anything you want during the non-fasting hours or days of the plan. These days are frequently referred to as "feasting" days by researchers.

Of course, continuing to consume harmful foods isn't the best approach to reap the advantages of intermittent fasting, but eliminating them on some days reduces your overall consumption. It might even give benefits in the long run.

• Has the Potential to Increase Life Expectancy

Longevity is one of the most often touted advantages of intermittent fasting. According to the National Institute on Aging, Rodent studies have demonstrated that when mice have put on regimens that severely restrict calories (typically during fasting times), many live longer and have fewer illnesses, including malignancies.

Is this advantage also available to humans? It does, according to those who advocate the diets. Long-term research, however, has failed to establish this advantage.

There have been observational studies relating religious fasting to long-term longevity advantages, according to a study published in 2010. It was difficult to say if the advantage came from fasting or if other variables were at play.

• Assists with weight loss

The authors of a review of intermittent fasting study published in 2018 say that the studies they looked at demonstrated a substantial reduction in fat mass among clinical trial participants.

They also discovered that intermittent fasting, regardless of BMI, was effective in weight loss (BMI). According to the report, researchers looked at short-term weight loss, but longer-term trials are needed.

Body Mass Index (BMI) is an out-of-date, skewed metric that ignores various characteristics, including body composition, ethnicity, race, gender, and age.

Despite its flaws, BMI is still commonly utilized in the medical field since it is a low-cost and rapid way to assess possible health status and consequences.

Intermittent fasting might not be any more successful than other calorie-restricting regimens. The weight reduction advantages of intermittent fasting and standard diets (defined as continuous calorie restriction) were equivalent in a 2018 study.

In a major meta-analysis published in 2018, researchers looked at 11 studies that lasted anywhere from 8 to 24 weeks. When it came to weight reduction and metabolic benefits, the authors of the study found that intermittent fasting and constant calorie restriction had equivalent outcomes. To conclude, longer trials are required.

It's also likely that weight reduction outcomes are influenced by age. The effects of intermittent fasting (time-restricted food) on young (20-year-old) vs. older (50-year-old) males were investigated in a research published in the journal Nutrition in 2018.

Intermittent fasting reduced body mass modestly in young men but not in older individuals. Muscle power, on the other hand, was similar in both groups.

• Glucose Management

Some intermittent fasting researchers reported in 2018 that this eating pattern could assist persons with type 2 diabetes regulate their blood sugar levels by causing weight reduction in overweight or obese people, but that it can decrease insulin sensitivity in others.

Over seven months, a case series published in 2018 proved the effectiveness of fasting (under medical supervision and with dietary instruction) in reversing insulin resistance while maintaining blood sugar management. Patients could quit using insulin, lose weight, shrink their waist circumference, and improve their blood glucose levels overall.

However, with a bigger sample size, research published in 2019 found a less striking influence on blood glucose management. In adults with type 2 diabetes, researchers conducted a 24-month follow-up of a 12-month study comparing intermittent fasting with continuous calorie restriction. HbA1c values increased in both groups, according to the researchers.

Other studies have found that, despite various dietary treatments, blood glucose levels in people with type 2 diabetes tend to rise with time, despite a variety of dietary interventions.

According to the study's authors, intermittent calorie restriction, rather than continuous energy restriction, could be beneficial for sustaining lower HbA1c levels. However, bigger sample sizes and further research are needed to validate the effect.

Other Health Advantages

Intermittent fasting has been linked to various health advantages in certain studies. However, almost every study states that further research is needed to completely comprehend the advantage.

Intermittent fasting during Ramadan, for example, was shown to lower total cholesterol, LDL cholesterol, and triglycerides in study participants, according to research published in

2018. A rise in HDL ("good") cholesterol levels was also beneficial to the subjects.

Another study discovered that intermittent fasting (particularly time-restricted meals) could successfully treat low-grade systemic inflammation and several age-related chronic illnesses associated with immune function without impairing physical performance. Only 40 males were investigated, and bigger variation research is required.

DISADVANTAGES

• Side Effects

According to studies looking into the advantages of intermittent fasting, certain negative effects can arise during the fasting period of the eating regimen. It's fairly unusual to feel irritable or weary or to have heartburn, constipation, dehydration, poor sleep quality, or anemia.

Intermittent fasting could be harmful if you have hypertension, high LDL cholesterol, excessively high uric acid levels in the blood, hyperglycemia, cardiovascular illness, or liver and kidney disease.

• Physical Activity Reduction

The lack of physical activity is perhaps one of the most noticeable negative effects. The majority of intermittent fasting programs do not include a physical exercise suggestion.

Unsurprisingly, many who adhere to the plans might get so exhausted that they fail to fulfill their daily step objectives and perhaps abandon their normal exercise routines. It's been suggested that more studies be done to understand how intermittent fasting affects physical activity habits.

• Extreme Hunger

In the fasting stage of an IF eating plan, it's not uncommon for people to feel extremely hungry. When they are among individuals eating regular meals and snacks, their hunger could become more intense.

• Medications

Many people who take drugs find that taking their prescription with meals helps lessen some adverse effects. Several drugs expressly state that they should be taken with meals. Therefore, taking drugs while fasting could be difficult.

Before beginning an IF program, anybody who takes medication should consult with their doctor to ensure that the fasting period will not interfere with the medicine's efficacy or negative effects.

• Nutritious Eating Isn't a Priority

Most intermittent fasting regimens focus on timing rather than meal selection. As a result, no foods are avoided (even those that are low in value), and those high in nutrition are not promoted. As a result, those who follow the diet are unlikely to learn how to consume healthy, balanced food.

It's unlikely that you'll acquire fundamental healthy eating and cooking skills while on a short-term intermittent fasting program, such as cooking with healthy oils, eating more veggies, and picking whole grains over processed grains.

• Could Encourage Overeating

Meal quantity and frequency are not regulated during many intermittent fasting methods' "feasting" stage. Instead, customers can eat as much as they want.

Unfortunately, this could encourage some people to overeat. If you feel starved after a day of total fasting, you could be tempted to overeat (or consume items high in fat, calories, salt, or added sugar) on days when "feasting" is permitted.

• Long-Term Constraints

While intermittent fasting is not new, much of the research studying the advantages of this eating strategy is relatively recent. As a result, it's difficult to say if the advantages will endure.

Furthermore, researchers frequently state that long-term studies are required to ascertain whether the eating plan is safe for more than a few months.

For the time being, the safest course of action is to choose and begin an IF regimen in consultation with your healthcare physician. Your provider can track your progress to verify that the eating style is healthy for you, including both advantages and problems.

LOSE WEIGHT

For many people, maintaining a healthy weight or decreasing excess body fat might get difficult as the years go by.

Weight gain after the age of 50 can be caused by unhealthy behaviors, a primarily sedentary lifestyle, poor food choices, and metabolic changes.

You can lose weight at any age, regardless of your medical conditions or physical ability, by making a few easy changes.

Here are the top 20 weight-loss strategies for those over 50.

1. Get into the habit of enjoying strength exercise.

Strength training is particularly crucial for older people, even if cardio receives a lot of emphasis on weight loss.

Sarcopenia is when your muscle mass decreases as you become older. Around the age of 50, muscle mass loss occurs, reducing your metabolism and contributing to weight gain.

After 50, your muscle mass reduces at roughly 12% per year, while your muscular strength declines at a rate of 1.5–5% per year.

So, including muscle-building activities in your workout program is critical for preventing age-related muscle loss and maintaining healthy body weight.

Strength training, such as weightlifting and bodyweight exercises can dramatically enhance muscular strength, size, and function.

Strength training can also help you lose weight by lowering body fat and increasing your metabolism, which can help you burn more calories throughout the day.

2. Form a group

It might be difficult to establish a healthy eating habit or exercise program. Sticking to your plan and accomplishing your wellness objectives could be easier if you team up with a friend, coworker, or family member.

For example, studies suggest that people who participate in weight-loss programs alongside friends are far more likely to keep their weight off in the long run.

Working out with friends can also help you stay committed to your fitness regimen and make it more fun.

3. Move more and sit less.

To lose extra body fat, you must burn more calories than you consume. That is why, while attempting to reduce weight, being more active throughout the day is critical.

Sitting at your desk for lengthy periods, for example, can sabotage your weight loss attempts. To combat this, even getting up from your desk and taking a five-minute stroll every hour will help you become more active at work.

According to studies, using a pedometer or Fitbit to count your steps can help you lose weight by boosting your activity and calorie expenditure.

Start with a reasonable step target based on your current activity levels using a pedometer or Fitbit. Then, progressively increase to 7,000–10,000 steps per day or more, depending on your general health.

4. Increase your protein consumption.

It is vital to get enough high-quality protein in your diet for weight reduction and prevent or reverse age-related muscle loss.

After 20, your resting metabolic rate (RMR), or the number of calories you burn at rest, declines by 1–2% every decade. This is linked to muscle loss as people become older.

On the other hand, a protein-rich diet can help prevent or reverse muscle loss. Increasing dietary protein has also been proved in several studies to help you lose weight and keep it off in the long run.

Furthermore, research reveals that older persons require more protein than younger adults, emphasizing the importance of including protein-rich foods in your snacks and meals.

5. Consult a dietician

Finding an eating pattern that promotes weight loss while still sustaining your body can be difficult.

Without needing to follow a rigorous diet, a qualified dietician can help you choose the most efficient technique for losing extra body fat. A nutritionist can also help you in lose weight by offering advice and support.

Working with a nutritionist to reduce weight can provide much better outcomes than trying it alone, according to research, but it might also help you maintain your weight reduction over time.

6. Prepare more meals at home

Several studies have shown that those who prepare and eat more meals at home have a healthier diet and weigh less than those who don't.

You have total control over what goes into — and what stays out of — your recipes when you cook them at home. It also allows you to test out new, healthy dishes that have caught your eye.

Start with preparing one or two meals at home each week if you dine out most of the time, and gradually build up this number until you are cooking at home more than you eat out.

7. Consume more vegetables and fruits

Fruits and vegetables are packed with nutrients that are vital to your health, and adding them to your diet is a simple, evidence-based way to drop excess weight.

According to a study of 10 research, increased daily vegetable consumption were linked to a 0.14-inch (0.36-cm) waist circumference reduction in women.

Another research found that consuming fruits and vegetables lowered body weight, waist circumference, and body fat in 26,340 women and men aged 35–65.

8. Engage the services of a personal trainer.

Working with a personal trainer could be especially beneficial for individuals new to working out since they can show you how to exercise properly to lose weight and avoid injury.

Personal trainers can also encourage you to exercise more by holding you accountable. They could even change your mind about working out.

10-week research of 129 participants found that 1 hour of one-on-one personal training enhanced exercise motivation and physical activity levels.

9. Reduce your reliance on convenience meals.

Consuming convenience meals such as fast food, sweets, and processed snacks have been linked to weight gain and could sabotage your weight reduction attempts.

Convenience foods are rich in calories and poor in critical elements such as protein, fiber, vitamins, and minerals. Fast food and other processed meals are sometimes referred to as "empty calories."

Cutting back on convenience foods and replacing them with nutrient-dense whole foods in healthful meals and snacks is a good strategy to reduce weight.

10. Find something you enjoy doing.

Finding a fitness plan that you can stick to for the long haul might be challenging. This is why it's critical to participate in things you like.

Sign up for a group activity like soccer or a running club, if you enjoy group activities. This will allow you to exercise with others.

If you like alone activities, go for a solo bike ride, a solo stroll, a solo hike, or a solo swim.

11. Have your health tested by a professional.

If you have trouble losing weight despite being active and eating a nutritious diet. In that case, you should rule out diseases that might make it difficult to lose weight, such as hypothyroidism and polycystic ovary syndrome (PCOS).

This is especially true if you have family members who suffer from these ailments.

Tell your doctor about your symptoms so he or she can choose the appropriate testing procedure to rule out any medical disorders that might be causing your weight loss problems.

12. Consume a diet rich in whole foods.

Following a diet rich in whole foods is one of the simplest methods to guarantee that your body receives the nutrients it requires to flourish.

Whole foods, such as vegetables, nuts, fruits, seeds, chicken, fish, legumes, and grains, are high in fiber, protein, and healthy fats, important for maintaining a healthy body weight.

In several studies, whole-food-based diets, both plant-based and those containing animal products, have been linked to weight loss.

13. Consume fewer calories at night.

Many studies have shown that consuming fewer calories at night can help you maintain a healthy weight and shed fat.

Over the course of six years, individuals who consumed more calories at supper were more than twice as likely to become obese as those who consumed more calories earlier in the day, according to a study of 1,245 adults.

Furthermore, individuals who consumed more calories at supper were more prone to developing metabolic syndrome, a combination of disorders that include elevated blood sugar and extra abdominal fat. Heart disease, diabetes, and stroke are all increased by metabolic syndrome.

Breakfast and lunch should include most of your calories, with a lighter dinner being a viable option for weight loss.

14. Pay attention to your body composition.

Although your body weight is an excellent measure of health, your body composition — the percentages of fat and fat-free mass in your body — is also significant.

Muscle mass, particularly in older persons, is a significant indicator of general health. Your objective should be to gain more muscle and lose extra fat.

There are several methods for calculating your body fat percentage. Measuring your waist, calves, chest, biceps, and thighs, on the other hand, can assist you in figuring out if you are losing fat and growing muscle.

15. Drink plenty of water in a healthy manner.

Drinks contain additional sugars and calories, such as sweetened coffee beverages, soda, juices, sports drinks, and pre-made smoothies.

Sugar-sweetened drinks, particularly those sweetened with high-fructose corn syrup, have been related to weight gain and obesity, diabetes, heart disease, and fatty liver disease.

Substituting healthy liquids like water and herbal tea for sugary beverages will help you lose weight and lower your chance of acquiring the chronic illnesses listed above.

16. Select the appropriate supplements

If you're tired and unmotivated, the correct vitamins might help you get the energy you need to achieve your objectives.

Your capacity to absorb some nutrients decreases as you get older, increasing your risk of deficiency. According to study, adults over 50, for example, are frequently lacking in folate and vitamin B12, two elements required for energy synthesis.

B vitamin deficiencies, such as B12 deficiency, can affect your mood, create tiredness, and prevent you from losing weight.

As a result, adults over the age of 50 should take a high-quality B-complex vitamin to help reduce the risk of insufficiency.

17. Keep added sugars to a minimum

Limiting foods high in added sugar for weight reduction at any age, such as sweetened drinks, sweets, cakes, cookies, ice cream, sweetened yogurts, and sugary cereals, is crucial.

Because sugar is added to so many meals, even things you wouldn't anticipate, like tomato sauce, salad dressing, and bread, reading the ingredient labels is the best way to find out if anything has sugar.

Look for "added sugars" on the nutrition information label or for typical sweeteners like cane sugar, high-fructose corn syrup, and agave in the ingredient list.

18. Improve the quality of your sleep

If you don't get enough decent sleep, your weight reduction efforts may be jeopardized. In multiple studies, sleep deprivation has been associated to an increased risk of obesity and has been proven to undermine weight loss attempts.

Those who slept 7 hours or more every night were 33 percent more likely to lose weight than those who slept less than 7 hours per night, according to a two-year study of 245 women. Better sleep quality was also associated to weight reduction success.

Aim for the recommended 7–9 hours of sleep every night, and increase the quality of your sleep by reducing light in your bedroom and avoiding using your phone or watching TV before bed.

19. Experiment with intermittent fasting.

IF is an eating pattern in which you only eat for a certain amount of time. The 16/8 approach, in which you eat for 8 hours and then fast for 16, is the most common intermittent fasting.

Intermittent fasting has been demonstrated to help people lose weight in several studies.

Furthermore, some test-tube and animal research shows that intermittent fasting could benefit older humans by extending life, reducing cell decline, and avoiding age-related alterations to mitochondria, your cells' energy-producing organelles.

20. Be more aware

Mindful eating is a simple method to enhance your connection with food while also helping you lose weight.

Mindful eating entails paying closer attention to what you eat and how you eat. It helps you understand your hunger and fullness cues and how food affects your mood and overall well-being.

Many studies have found that practicing mindful eating practices helps people lose weight and improve their eating habits.

There are no hard and fast rules for mindful eating, but eating slowly, paying attention to the scent and flavor of each mouthful, and keeping track of how you feel throughout meals are all simple methods to start.

Though weight reduction might become more difficult as you get older, several evidence-based treatments can help you attain and maintain a healthy body weight after 50.

Cutting added sugars from your diet, including strength training in your exercises, eating more protein, preparing meals at home, and eating a whole-food-based diet are just a few ways you can enhance your general health and shed excess body fat.

Try the suggestions above, and you'll find that losing weight after 50 is a snap.

BETTER SLEEP

You could drink a double latte at 9 p.m., sleep through your alarm, and wake up at midday when you were 20. Your connection with sleep has grown a lot more...dysfunctional now that you're over 40. You are up at least twice to pee if it takes you an hour to fall asleep, and you are awake for no reason around three a.m. If this describes you, know that you are not alone.

According to sleep expert Matthew Walker, author of Why We Sleep, the quality of sleep we obtain degrades as we get older due to a steady accumulation of the protein beta amyloid in the brain. He noted on Fresh Air that "the brain is not capable of creating the sleep that it still requires and the body still needs." However, while the decrease may start in your forties, it is not yet complete. "By the time you're in your forties, you've probably lost around 40 to 50 percent of the deep sleep you had when you were a teenager, for example." By the age of 70, you could have lost about 90% of your deep sleep." Eep.

So, what are we going to do about it? While we can't stop time (unless you're Kerry Washington), there are a few sleep expert-approved methods for ladies over ffity to fall asleep faster...and stay asleep longer.

1. Make A 'Last Call' On Liquids For Yourself.

You're well aware of the importance of staying hydrated. However, if you're getting up many times a night to pee, it's time to give your bladder a nighttime curfew. "As women age, their pelvic floor muscles atrophy and their vaginal tissue thins, making it tougher to manage urine desires at night," says Dr. Joshua Tal, Idle Group's Sleep Advisor. Women over fifty should cease consuming liquids two hours before night, according to him. While caffeine and alcohol are particularly disruptive to sleep, even water can trigger wake-ups in the middle of the night, disrupting your sleep patterns.

2. Lower The Thermostat (Like, Much Lower Than You Think)

Hey, you, with the thermostat set at 74 degrees in your bedroom. The pleasant ambiance in your room could be interfering with your sleep. "Your body needs to cool down to go asleep, which is why it's usually easier to fall asleep in a room that's too chilly than in one that's too hot," Walker explains. To obtain the best night's sleep, he suggests putting your thermostat between 65 and 68 degrees. (If that seems terribly cold, he doesn't suggest curling up under a giant duvet and wearing flannel PJs.)

3. Get Out Of Your Head

Have you ever heard of the term "invisible workload"? If you have a partner, children, a job, elderly relatives, or all of the above, you probably spend time arranging your thoughts before going to bed. (By "organizing," we mean generating a million mental to-do lists, figuring out what to pack for the kids' lunches tomorrow, deconstructing that strange phone chat with your boss, and brainstorming what to gift your mother for her birthday in three months.) This is referred to as "emotional labor." "Many of my over-40 female clients tell me that as soon as they get into bed, their minds fly over their to-do lists, reviewing the day's accomplishments and disappointments or planning for tomorrow," adds Dr. Tal. Yep. That reminds me of something. What is the issue? You've started to associate your bed with work rather than sleep. To cleanse your thoughts, Dr. Tal recommends getting out of bed and writing down all of your anxieties.

4. Take A Shot Of Melatonin

If you're having trouble sleeping, your first reaction might be to seek a prescription sleep medication from your doctor. However, according to Walker, sleep aids don't actually help you sleep. They are sedatives, so while you will be drugged for the night, you will not be getting the rest you require. Walker recommends using melatonin supplements for elderly individuals who have a lower natural melatonin output. Melatonin is a substance that helps you adjust the timing of your sleep, while it isn't officially a sleep aid. "A whole slew of various chemicals and brain systems really create sleep and bring you into sleep," explains walker. "Melatonin just predicts when you'll go asleep, not that you'll fall asleep." Still, if you've seen a reduction in the quality of your sleep over time, it's worth a try.

5. Remember To Pay Attention To Your Nose.

If you're anything like us, you wake up most mornings with a cement-filled nose, especially in the winter. Dr. Tal adds, "Laying down horizontally increases blood flow and mucous to the nose, causing discomfort and disrupting sleep." "A humidifier can assist with this problem at night, but make sure it's clean so it doesn't circulate mold and mildew." If your congestion persists, he recommends replacing your present mattress with an Eden Mattress, which is hypoallergenic and created with organic materials.

6. Perform A Sleep Hygiene Analysis

You spend seven hours in bed, but are you receiving the best possible sleep? According to Dr. Lisa Medalie, PsyD, CBSM, a behavioral sleep medicine specialist, it's time to undertake a sleep audit. Do your windows have hefty blackout shades? Do you sleep in PJs that are both comfortable and breathable? Is it possible that noise from the street or the flat above you is waking you up? Examine your nighttime routine next. Before going to bed, did you watch TV or check your email? Do you want to have a glass of wine? Do you want to eat something that contains chocolate? Any one of these seemingly innocuous behaviors might be keeping you up at night.

7. Experiment With Square Breathing

You must assist you in relaxing into a deep sleep. We attempt square breathing when we're having one of those "tossing and turning" nights. Basically, you use your diaphragm to breathe in and out for four counts:

For a count of four, inhale through your nose (1, 2, 3, 4)

Hold your breath for four counts (1, 2, 3, 4)

For a count of four, exhale through your mouth (1, 2, 3, 4)

For a count of four, pause and hold (1, 2, 3, 4)

Repeat as needed until you've drifted off to sleep.

A HEALTHY HEART

You've probably figured out what kind of food plan makes you feel the best, and you've tried enough various sorts of workouts to know what you genuinely enjoy doing.

In some respects, though, it can be more difficult. Menopause causes your body to change in ways that aren't always pleasant. You could get more out of breath undertaking an exercise that you used to love a few years ago. Perhaps new concerns have arisen, such as bone loss or maintaining a healthy heart. The latter is a common complaint among women over 50, according to cardiologists.

Cardiologists Harvey Kramer, MD, and Matthew Budoff, MD, both said they talk to all of their female patients over 50 about heart health. Here, they share what they are so you can live by them, too.

According to cardiologists, good heart health for women over 50 begins with four important fundamentals:

1. Make sure your heart is in good shape to begin with.

If you have any worries about your heart or haven't had a checkup in a while, Dr. Kramer, who works with Nuvance Health, recommends scheduling an appointment with your doctor. "Your physician should analyze your risk for heart disease during your health assessment to ensure that your heart is healthy and to detect any danger of developing heart disease in the future," Dr. Kramer advises. "A physical examination should include a medical history, blood pressure check, and heart exam, as well as an electrocardiogram (ECG) and test work to establish blood sugar levels and lipid profile." (You can also use the American Heart Association's risk assessor to determine your risk of heart disease.)

According to Dr. Kramer, if your examination reveals any health concerns, such as high blood pressure or high blood sugar levels, the next step is to speak with your doctor about handling them. He claims that it all starts with one's lifestyle choices, such as finding methods to consume nutritious meals that he enjoys and being active. Medications, however, can play a role depending on the severity of the difficulties.

2. Exercising for at least 150 minutes each week is recommended.

Both cardiologists said they constantly stress the necessity of mobility to their patients, particularly those over 50. (After all, their job description includes the term cardio.) Dr. Budoff adds, "Exercise is essential for women over 50 since it helps with cognition, heart disease, and bone strength, which is extremely important as we age." According to Dr. Kramer, a decent rule of thumb is to exercise for 150 minutes of moderate physical activity every week.

3. Create a network of people who can help you.

Dr. Kramer understands that altering your lifestyle isn't always simple, especially if you're not used to exercising for 150 minutes a week or attempting to eat healthier. This is why he believes that having a support system might be beneficial. Scheduling a nightly phone call with a pal, during which you both catch up while strolling around your different areas, is one suggestion. Perhaps you and your partner enjoy healthy cooking competitions at home. It might also look for a community online. "There are online programs that can help you improve your behaviors," says Dr. Kramer.

4. Increase your garlic consumption.

Garlic is a favorite of Dr. Budoff's, not just because it enhances the flavor of food. "Old garlic extract appears to have the single greatest impact on heart health of any known dietary supplement," he says. "It promotes healthy blood pressure and lowers bad cholesterol levels, decreases plaque in coronary arteries, and enhances the health of blood vessel walls," according to research.

5. Check to see whether you're receiving adequate rest.

One of the most crucial heart health recommendations for women over 50? Getting adequate sleep is essential. "We all know that getting enough sleep enables the body to heal itself. A healthy heart necessitates a good night's sleep, "According to Dr. Budoff. He says that not receiving enough puts you at risk for cardiovascular and coronary health problems. According to the National Sleep Foundation, adults, particularly those in their 50s, should obtain seven to nine hours of sleep every night. According to the National Sleep Foundation, women have greater sleeping issues than males, and one cause for this is stress. As a result, finding methods to alleviate stress is essential.

6. Brush and floss at least once a day.

You might believe that your mouth has little to do with your cardiovascular health, but according to Dr. Budoff, they do. "Several studies have found that oral and heart health are linked," he explains. "When germs in your mouth are discharged into your circulation, they can cause inflammation and artery stiffness, potentially leading to heart attack and stroke." Brushing and flossing every day is undoubtedly a good idea, especially if you're consuming a lot of garlic.

According to Dr. Kramer, the actual goal is to make these health principles ones that you follow to the point that they're thoroughly interwoven into your everyday life. However, he advises not to feel terrible if one slips by the wayside. "It's tough to change habits, let alone improve your lifestyle," he adds. "If you fail to change your behaviors, try again. This could take several attempts until you master your new way of living."

Chapter 5: INTERMITTENT FASTING MINDSET

For many individuals, reducing weight is fighting against themselves: their form, their weaker self, and their own body.

After all, it appears to be common sense that everything boils down to discipline and adhering to the "no pain, no gain" approach. We forget that our bodies are not machines when we think like this. Our bodies stop working correctly due to all the stress we put on ourselves.

What is the solution? The appropriate frame of mind!

This chapter will discover why your thinking is so crucial to losing weight. Also, how intermittent fasting might aid in the development of a more optimistic mindset.

What role do your thoughts have in your weight reduction success?

Have you ever failed to achieve your weight-loss objectives? Have you had to cope with insensitive remarks regarding your weight? That is precisely what has a bad impact on your thinking. Sure, you want to get it right the first time and eventually succeed. As a result, you put yourself under a lot of stress.

When it comes to reducing weight, stress is the biggest deterrent.

According to studies, too much stress might prevent fat burning. This is mostly due to the stress chemicals generated, such as cortisol, which inhibits fat metabolism.

But you have the power to alter your mental state! You have the power to affect and change it - if you so want!

Now is the time to change your thinking.

This might take some practice, but remembering these concepts is extremely important:

1. Make an invitation to your body.

2. Don't try to oppose it.

3. Develop the ability to pay attention to your body's requirements. Patience is required.

4. Recognize and respect its limitations; don't push yourself too hard if you don't feel like it.

You'll notice that everything changes once you stop thinking of your body as the adversary! Many things get simpler when you work WITH it rather than against it.

How intermittent fasting aids in the development of a more optimistic outlook

Intermittent fasting can aid in the development of a more cheerful attitude. Fasting on a regular basis enhances your connection with food (and with yourself).

You relearn how to listen to your own needs.

You grow more conscious and autonomous by removing yourself from the steady stream of consumption.

While fasting, you give your body the time and space to recuperate and renew.

Weight loss does not have to be a struggle.

The secret to your success has the appropriate mindset and attitude. Isn't it true that it's much easier stated than done? Yes, it is! Even so, it's well worth it.

One thing to keep in mind is that changing your perspective takes time. If you find yourself reverting to previous habits, don't become discouraged. Keep a good attitude and keep going - even if you're intermittent fasting! After some time, you'll notice that it happens less frequently. You're getting closer to your objective with each step! You've got this!

Chapter 6: INTERMITTENT FASTING AND EXERCISE

In today's wellness world, there are many different meal plans available to assist you in achieving your fitness objectives. Intermittent fasting has become one of the most popular diets, and its relative simplicity has helped it grow in popularity. However, a well-known reality is that a healthy eating pattern is only one-half of the puzzle. Combining a balanced eating plan with frequent physical activity is vital to get the best outcomes. Is this plan, however, appropriate for all diets? Is working exercise with intermittent fasting compatible? Is it going to be good for your overall health?

Intermittent fasting is a popular meal plan whose foundation is self-evident: dieters must fast for specific periods. This is dependent on the type of intermittent fasting people choose. Some people prefer 5:2 fasting (fasting only two days each week), while others only fast once or twice a month. One of the most prevalent concepts is 16:8. You should eat all of your meals during an 8-hour window each day and fast for the remaining 16 hours. This is a common version because these 16 hours generally include sleep time. You don't have to have breakfast and can eat whenever you want until a particular hour in the evening.

No official food lists specify what you should and should not eat; your meal plan is entirely up to you. If you're fasting to lose weight, it's critical to select good food choices and keep track of your portions. You'll only be able to lose or maintain a healthy weight this way. Aside from that, your body has nutritional requirements, and your daily menu should help you meet those requirements.

Many people believe that weight reduction is an efficient technique to combat obesity and reduce calorie intake over time. There are, however, certain disadvantages. For example, during the non-fasting phase, some individuals could experience overeating or binge eating. During their non-fasting phase, many people choose to eat unhealthy things.

More scientific evidence is needed to support the intermittent fasting method's effectiveness and safety. Despite this, many individuals use it for dieting and are pleased with the outcomes. If you want to try this weight reduction method, you should first talk to your doctor to ensure you can do it safely.

Is It Possible to Exercise While Intermittent Fasting?

As you can see, the fundamental principle is to avoid eating for an extended time. You also understand that your body needs nourishment for any activity, particularly exercise. Is it feasible to mix intermittent fasting and exercise without causing harm to your health?

The material on this subject is highly contradictory. It's critical to think about your general health, exercise level, age, lifestyle, and dietary habits. That is why you should seek the advice of a medical expert.

First and foremost, folks who prioritize working out should choose a diet that will supply fuel to their bodies. Physical activity puts your body under stress, and if it doesn't get enough calories, the tension becomes even worse. It is also possible that your body will start breaking down your muscle mass for energy if it can't acquire it from the meal you ate due to a shortage of fuel. People who combine intermittent fasting and exercise might experience a lack of energy and find it more difficult to complete their workouts. It's also possible to have a slowed metabolic rate.

However, there are certain advantages, such as increased fat burning and weight loss. Let's look at the risks and advantages of combining intermittent fasting with exercise.

The Advantages and Disadvantages of Intermittent Fasting and Exercise

The advantages and disadvantages of combining intermittent fasting and exercise are listed below.

PROS

Unwanted Pounds Can Be Peeled Off

Your body will most likely use its glycogen stores for energy throughout your fasting days (or hours). When they are exhausted, the body begins to burn body fat for energy and fuel.

People who exercise while fasting burn more fat during exercise than those who exercise after eating a meal, according to one meta-analysis (4)

The data on the influence on weight loss, on the other hand, is a little murky.

Another study found that people who exercised while hungry had no better long-term weight loss results than those who ate a meal before training sessions.

It has anti-aging properties.

According to one study, combining intermittent fasting with physical activity can help to slow down the aging process and reduce illness risks. The alterations in metabolism that this combination could generate are responsible for this impact, albeit research in this area is still in its early stages.

The Autophagy Process Can Be Boosted

This is a bodily mechanism that aids in removing damaged body cells and organelles to replace them with healthy ones. According to a a preliminary study, combining intermittent fasting with exercise can help speed up this process.

CONS

Muscle Growth Could Be More Difficult

According to research, intermittent research, intermittent fasting can cause people to build less muscle mass than those who follow a regular eating routine without calorie restriction. They could, however, preserve greater muscle mass than individuals who restrict calories daily.

It has an impact on your blood sugar and blood pressure levels.

Intermittent fasting combined with exercise can lower blood sugar levels. Blood sugar levels that are too low might induce fainting. Low blood pressure and lightheadedness are also possible side effects.

This could result in poor performance.

According to studies, exercising without enough nutrition might result in poor performance, particularly among trained athletes.

How To Work Out While Fasting

Here are a few suggestions to help you stay healthy and achieve your exercise goals:

• If you're a beginner, it's best to stick to low-intensity workouts. You won't be short of energy this way.

• Paying attention to what your body is trying to tell you is crucial. This is critical since you might begin to feel ill throughout your workouts. You can avoid injuries and various health problems if you pay attention to yourself.

• It's critical to keep hydrated, including during fasting, eating periods, and workouts. You'll be able to replenish the fluids your body loses while exercising in this manner. On fasting days, drink much more water. Certain coconut water or other electrolyte-containing liquids can assist in replacing your body's electrolyte levels, but if you're fasting, you should avoid those with sugar.

• Think about the sort of fasting you're doing. The lesser the intensity of your exercises should be, the longer you are fasting.

• Keep track of the relationship between your exercises and macronutrients. If you choose strength exercise, your body will require more carbohydrates. Carbs are used less in high-intensity interval training and other aerobic activities.

• If you choose to exercise weights, it could be best to do so within your eating window and then follow up with high-protein meals to maintain and assist increase muscle mass.

• Always talk to your doctor about your plans.

What Are The Best Intermittent Fasting Exercises?

Everything in this scenario is dependent on the type of intermittent fasting you pick. You could do both strength and aerobic training if you follow a 16:8 diet. If you wish to practice alternate days or 24-hour fasting and continue exercising on the fasting days, you should choose less intense workouts. Yoga and pilates will be excellent choices. Walking is also acceptable.

When Is It Better To Work Out On Intermittent Fasting?

• Fasting Intermittently And Working Out In The Morning

This is probably the best option, as it will help you maintain your circadian rhythm. It's also possible that doing your exercises at the end of your fasting period will allow you to eat later. It will be difficult to exercise after a long period of fasting at first, but you will get used to it. You can change the intensity of your workout depending on how your body is feeling.

• Intermittent fasting and nighttime workouts

Training sessions that are scheduled too close to bedtime are not recommended, as they often reduce the quality of your sleep.

BENEFITS OF EXERCISE

Exercise is one of the most important activities for older adults to maintain independence.

Despite this, it is common for people to become increasingly sedentary as they become older.

Staying active and healthy for as long as possible will help you be happier and live a better life. So, in this chapter, we'll look at the specific advantages of moving more.

1. Maintains independence - This is possibly the most important advantage of exercising as you become older. While care homes are necessary for some elderly persons, many would like to remain in their own homes for as long as feasible. It's critical to stick to a workout routine that promotes this way of life.

2. Improved cardiovascular health - Physical exercise decreases the risk of cardiovascular disease by 35% in adults and older persons. Heart attacks and strokes are medical illnesses that can have life-altering repercussions if they are survived. As a result, exercise can be a very effective preventive measure.

3. Can help with cognitive function - Dementia affects many older folks, with the Alzheimer's Society estimating that over 1 million people will have the disease by 2025. Exercise has been mentioned in certain research to assist minimize the disease's occurrence.

4. Lowers anxiety and depression — Many older persons can experience social isolation, disease, or disability, leading to mental health problems. Exercise provides several cognitive advantages, including decreasing anxiety and depression and a lower rate of relapse compared to other therapies.

5. Improves flexibility - Osteoarthritis causes stiffness and immobility in joints and muscles, making it difficult for elderly people to move around. While an exercise program won't be able to cure all age-related joint changes, it will help to keep muscles and joints moving.

6. Strengthens muscles - Muscles waste without activity. Similarly to how movement increases flexibility, resistance training develops key muscle groups to keep you mobile on your own. This is especially important while transitioning from sitting to standing, climbing and descending stairs, or walking.

7. Increases bone density — Many elderly people suffer from osteoporosis, in which bones weaken and become more prone to fractures. Resistance exercise has been shown to help preserve bone strength in older years.

8. Prevents falls - When people lose flexibility, strength, and coordination, they are in danger of falling. Illness or disability are two other possible risk factors. Exercise can help you avoid falling, being hurt, and going to the hospital.

9. Maintains hobbies - Losing one's capacity to participate in activities due to inactivity can have both physical and psychological consequences. Hobbies are necessary for staying socially connected and active in life.

10. Assists with weight loss – Diet and inactivity can lead to weight gain in later years, leading to an increased risk of medical conditions. Exercise is not only a calorie-burning activity, but it can also motivate you to eat better. Furthermore, physical activity has been shown to reduce the risk of Type 2 Diabetes by up to 40%.

Behavioral scientists have shown exercise to enable other productive routines, such as healthy eating and social interaction. As a result, physical exercise can have favorable side effects.

12. Improves sleep — Getting adequate sleep has been shown to prevent the occurrence of chronic physical and mental health disorders, making it critical for our emotional well-being. Exercise can help you sleep better by reducing mental activity and inducing physical weariness.

13. Maintains social relationships — Exercising in a social setting holds you accountable and is also highly satisfying. Whether it is a daily stroll in the park with a buddy or an exercise class at the local leisure center, maintaining social relationships is important for maintaining good health in older years.

14. Improves confidence — Regular movement and training can enhance confidence by nurturing the mind-body link and

the physical advantages of exercise. Furthermore, increased self-esteem gained via exercise can increase happiness and a superior quality of life in later years.

15. Increases lifetime — Research has shown that regular exercise can increase life expectancy by 3-5 years. Physical activity extends one's life and enhances the quality of that life.

16. It's a lot of fun! Why do kids enjoy playing games? They don't think about the health advantages of exercise; instead, they see movement as a pleasure in and of itself. Although returning to exercise after a lengthy layoff could be difficult at first, you'll quickly appreciate the benefits as your fitness and mobility improve.

Before exercising, talk to your doctor or a physiotherapist if you have a medical problem or are unclear about what form of physical exercise is right.

Furthermore, to avoid damage, it's best to start slowly and allow your body to adjust to a new level of exercise.

FAQs

• Can I Exercise While Intermittent Fasting?

There are no specific guidelines in this area. Everything is dependent on your fitness level, the sort of workouts you pick, and whether or not you practice intermittent fasting. You should take a break if you feel lightheaded or dizzy throughout your workout.

• What Is The Best Food To Eat After A Workout To Break A Fast?

People who follow an intermittent fasting diet often eat less food. This is why it's so important to eat super-nutritious and healthful meals throughout your non-fasting phase. Even though there are no hard and fast rules on what meals you can eat within your eating window, you should be careful. It is advisable to choose healthy foods to reduce weight and improve your health. The best choices will be fruits and vegetables, lean cuts of meat, whole grains, and other healthful meals. Protein and carbohydrates are required for muscle growth and recovery. Your calorie intake and amount are determined by various factors, including your fitness objectives. You can utilize internet calculators or talk to a certified dietician (which is preferable) to figure this out.

• Is It Possible To Do Keto Intermittent Fasting And Workout?

The guidelines are essentially the same as for a conventional intermittent fasting diet. However, you should use caution when combining the keto and intermittent fasting diets. You shouldn't start both weight-loss methods at the same time, as such drastic lifestyle changes put a lot of strain on your body. It takes at least a few weeks to become acclimated to such changes. You should start with the keto diet and then go to intermittent fasting. Your body will gradually adjust to the alterations in your diet in this manner.

If you are experiencing weariness, nausea, dizziness, mental fog, or injuries, it is best to discontinue your diet and consult your doctor. The same is true if you require a significant amount of time to recuperate from your workout sessions. Because of the keto diet, it is a significant struggle for your body to go without meals for an extended length of time and to avoid certain food categories. This, when combined with exercise, can lead to various health problems.

As you can see, intermittent fasting and exercise can complement one another. When it comes to time and type of workouts, you need to be extremely cautious. Make sure they aren't too difficult for you and comfortable with them. Remember to choose nutritious foods that will replenish your body and help it work properly. Carry out your workouts safely and correctly, selecting them based on your fitness level and paying attention to your body. Make it a habit to hydrate your body as often as possible and in the appropriate proportions. Healthy, high-quality sleep is essential not just for your health but also for achieving your weight-loss objectives. Before you begin your intermittent fasting adventure and pick certain workouts, you should consult with your healthcare provider. Maintain your health by taking care of yourself.

Chapter 7: INTERMITTENT FASTING AND DIET

Calorie restriction has been found in animals to extend their longevity and enhance their tolerance to different metabolic stressors. Although there is significant support for calorie restriction in animal research, the data in human studies are less persuasive. Diet supporters think that the stress of intermittent fasting triggers an immunological response that heals cells while also causing favorable metabolic changes (reduction in triglycerides, LDL cholesterol, blood pressure, weight, fat mass, blood glucose). This diet's supporters are concerned that they could overeat on non-fasting days to make up for calories lost during fasting. However, when compared to other weight loss approaches, research has demonstrated that this is not the case. Intermittent fasting was found to be helpful for weight reduction in a comprehensive evaluation of 40 research, with an average loss of 7-11 pounds over 10 weeks. The investigations varied greatly in size and length of follow-up, ranging from 4 to 334 patients and 2 to 104 weeks. It's worth noting that diverse study designs and intermittent fasting strategies were utilized as participant characteristics (lean vs. obese). The fasting group was compared to a comparison group and/or a control group (either continuous calorie restriction or ordinary lifestyle) in half of the studies, while the other half looked at an intermittent fasting group alone in the other half. Here's a quick rundown of what they discovered:

• The percentage of students that dropped out ranged from 0 to 65 percent. There were no significant differences in dropout rates between the fasting and continuous calorie restriction groups. Overall, the study found that intermittent fasting did not have a low dropout rate, implying that it was not necessarily simpler to stick to than other weight management methods.

• There was no significant difference in weight reduction or body composition changes between the 12 clinical studies that compared the fasting and the continuous calorie restriction groups.

• Despite considerable weight reduction and lower leptin hormone levels, the intermittent fasting groups did not exhibit an overall increase in hunger in 10 trials that looked at appetite changes (a hormone that suppresses appetite).

Intermittent fasting was not shown to be more successful than daily calorie restriction in a randomized controlled experiment that tracked 100 obese people for a year. Subjects were placed on an alternating day fast (alternating days of one meal of 25% of baseline calories versus 125 percent of baseline calories divided over three meals) or daily calorie restriction (75 percent of baseline calories divided over three meals) for the 6-month weight-loss phase, as recommended by the American Heart Association. After 6 months, both groups' calorie amounts were raised by 25% with the objective of weight maintenance. The groups' participants shared comparable features, with most of them being women and in good health. Weight loss, compliance rates, and cardiovascular risk factors were all investigated in the study. When they compared the two groups, they discovered the following:

• There were no significant variations in body composition, weight loss, or rebound (e.g., fat mass, lean mass).

• Blood pressure, fasting glucose, heart rate, and fasting insulin did not change significantly. Despite no changes in total cholesterol or triglycerides after 12 months, the alternate-day fasting group had considerably higher LDL cholesterol levels. The authors made no mention of a potential reason.

• The alternate-day fasting group had a greater dropout rate (38%) than the daily calorie restriction group (29 percent). On non-fasting days, participants in the fasting group ate less food than advised, but they ate more food than suggested on fasting days.

Pitfalls to Avoid

This type of diet would be difficult for someone who eats every few hours (e.g., snacks between meals, grazes). It would also be inappropriate for persons with diseases like diabetes, which necessitate eating at regular intervals owing to metabolic changes caused by their drugs. When food is reintroduced after a lengthy period of food deprivation or semi-starvation, one is in danger of overeating, leading to undesirable habits, including an increased preoccupation with food.

Intermittent fasting should be avoided by people who have the following conditions:

• Diabetes

- Self-restriction illnesses including unhealthy self-restriction (anorexia or bulimia nervosa)

- Medications that necessitate food intake

- Adolescents are in an active growing stage.

- Pregnancy and lactation

Unanswered Questions

- How frequently and for how long should one fast to experience therapeutic results?

- Is this diet safe and good for everyone (e.g., the general public, people with chronic conditions at higher risk, the elderly)?

- How does intermittent fasting affect your health in the long run?

- Is there a danger of negatively influencing other family members' eating habits, particularly in youngsters who watch their parents fasting and missing meals?

Although animal studies have shown some advantages of calorie restriction, no corresponding benefits of intermittent fasting have been reported in people. In terms of weight reduction, biochemical changes, compliance rates, and decreased hunger, it is uncertain if intermittent fasting is preferable to other weight management approaches. Certain persons who eat only one or two meals each day or do not eat for lengthy periods are more likely to stick to this diet.

Further high-quality research, including randomized controlled trials with more than one year of follow-up, is needed to prove a direct effect and the potential advantages of intermittent fasting. At this time, no firm advice on intermittent fasting for weight loss can be offered.

MEDITERRANEAN DIET

The Mediterranean diet is based on the traditional cuisine that people in Mediterranean nations like France, Spain, Greece, and Italy consume.

According to the researchers, the patients in this study were extremely healthy and had a minimal chance of developing a variety of chronic diseases.

Although there are no particular dietary guidelines, fruits, vegetables, whole grains, legumes, nuts, seeds, and heart-healthy fats are often encouraged. Refined cereals, processed meals, and added sugar should all be avoided.

A body of evidence suggests that the Mediterranean diet can help people lose weight and avoid heart attacks, strokes, type 2 diabetes, and premature mortality.

As a result, the Mediterranean diet is frequently suggested to those who want to enhance their health and protect themselves against chronic illness.

Benefits

An extensive number of health advantages have been connected to the Mediterranean diet.

It is good for your heart.

The Mediterranean diet's capacity to boost heart health has been thoroughly researched.

Studies have linked the Mediterranean diet to a reduced risk of heart disease and stroke.

One research compared the Mediterranean diet to a low-fat diet and found that the Mediterranean diet was more successful at slowing plaque development in the arteries, which is a key risk factor for heart disease.

According to other studies, the Mediterranean diet can help reduce diastolic and systolic blood pressure, which is good for heart health.

Helps to maintain a healthy blood sugar level

Vegetables, nuts, fruits, seeds, whole grains, and heart-healthy fats are all encouraged in the Mediterranean diet.

As a result, adhering to this eating pattern can aid in the stabilization of blood sugar levels and prevent type 2 diabetes.

Multiple studies have discovered that following a Mediterranean diet can lower fasting blood sugar levels and enhance hemoglobin A1C levels, a test used to assess long-term blood sugar control.

Insulin resistance, a disorder in which the body's capacity to use insulin to efficiently manage blood sugar levels is impaired, has also been linked to the Mediterranean diet.

Protects brain function

Several studies suggest that the Mediterranean diet is good for your brain and might prevent you from cognitive loss as you age.

For example, adherence to the Mediterranean diet was linked to enhanced memory and lower levels of numerous risk factors for Alzheimer's disease in research, including 512 persons.

In other studies, the Mediterranean diet has also been linked to a decreased risk of dementia, cognitive impairment, and Alzheimer's disease.

Furthermore, adopting the Mediterranean diet was connected to gains in cognitive function, memory, attention, and processing speed in healthy older persons.

What is the best way to follow it?

Healthy foods include vegetables, seeds, legumes, fruits, nuts, potatoes, whole grains, fish, seafood, herbs, spices, and extra virgin olive oil.

Consumption of poultry, cheese, eggs, and yogurt should be limited.

Moderate consumption of red meat, sugar-sweetened beverages, added sugars, processed meat, refined oils, refined grains, and other highly processed foods is recommended.

Foods to consume

It's debatable whether foods fit the Mediterranean diet, partially because there are differences across nations.

Most research focused on a plant-based diet that was low in animal products and meat. However, it is recommended that you consume fish and seafood at least twice a week.

Mediterranean lifestyle includes regular physical exercise, sharing meals with others, and reducing stress.

Fruits and vegetables may be used fresh, frozen, dried, or canned, but check package labels for added sugar and salt.

The following healthy Mediterranean foods should be included in your diet:

Carrots, tomatoes, broccoli, kale, spinach, onions, cauliflower, Brussels sprouts, cucumbers, potatoes, sweet potatoes, turnips.

Fruits include apples, bananas, oranges, pears, strawberries, grapes, dates, figs, melons, and peaches.

Macadamia nuts, hazelnuts, almonds, walnuts, cashews, almond butter, and peanut butter are nuts, sunflower seeds, pumpkin seeds, seeds, and nut butter.

Pulses, beans, lentils, peas, chickpeas, and peanuts are examples of legumes.

Whole grains include Oats, brown rice, rye, barley, maize, buckwheat, whole wheat bread, and pasta.

Trout, tuna, mackerel, salmon, sardines, shrimp, crab, oysters, clams, and mussels are examples of fish and seafood.

Chicken, duck, and turkey are examples of poultry.

Chicken, quail, and duck eggs.

Dairy products include cheese, milk, and yogurt.

Mint, rosemary, sage, garlic, basil, cinnamon, nutmeg, and pepper are some of the herbs and spices used.

Extra virgin olive oil, avocados, olives, and avocado oil are all good sources of healthy fats.

Foods to stay away from

When following the Mediterranean diet, you should avoid the following processed foods and ingredients:

Added sugar can be found in various meals, but it is particularly prevalent in soda, sweets, syrup, table sugar, ice cream, and baked goods.

Refined grains include spaghetti, tortillas, chips, white bread, and crackers.

Fried meals, margarine, and other processed foods contain trans fats.

Refined oils include soybean oil, canola oil, cottonseed oil, and grapeseed oil.

Meat that has been processed, such as hot dogs, sausages, deli meats, and beef jerky

Highly processed foods include fast food, convenience meals, microwave popcorn, and granola bars.

Beverages

On a Mediterranean diet, water should be your primary beverage.

This diet also includes a small quantity of red wine each day — perhaps one glass.

This is, however, entirely voluntary, and wine should be avoided by some individuals, such as those who are pregnant, have trouble drinking in moderation, or are on certain drugs that could interact with alcohol.

On the Mediterranean diet, coffee and tea are also healthful beverage options. Be wary of using a lot of extra sugar or cream.

Sugar-sweetened drinks, such as soda or sweet tea, are rich in added sugar and should be avoided. Fruit juice is OK in moderation, but you're better off eating entire fruits to obtain the fiber benefit.

Nutritious Snacks

If you become hungry in between meals, there are lots of healthy snack alternatives available on the Mediterranean diet.

Here are few suggestions to get you started:

a pound of nuts

a serving of fruit

Hummus-dressed baby carrots

a mixture of berries

grapes

Greek Yogurt

salt and pepper hard-boiled egg

pieces of apple with almond butter

guacamole and chopped bell peppers

fresh fruit with cottage cheese

Chia pudding

Eating Out

Many restaurant menu items are Mediterranean-friendly. Choose whole grains, veggies, legumes, fish, and healthy fats. It is also important to eat and relish your dinner with nice company, so choose something that sounds delicious.

Here are a few pointers to help you adjust foods while dining out:

As the main course, go for fish or seafood.

Inquire with your waitress whether your meal can be prepared using extra virgin olive oil.

Instead of butter, use olive oil on whole-grain toast.

Vegetables can be added to your order.

This restaurant eating-healthy advice could also be useful.

List of things to buy

Shopping around the store's periphery, where the whole foods are often available, is always a smart idea.

Choose nutrient-dense foods, including fruits, vegetables, nuts, seeds, legumes, and whole grains.

Here are some essentials for a Mediterranean diet shopping list:

Carrots, onions, broccoli, spinach, kale, garlic, zucchini, and mushrooms are examples of vegetables.

Peas, carrots, broccoli, and mixed vegetables (frozen)

Potatoes, yams, and sweet potatoes are examples of tubers.

Oranges, grapes, melons, apples, bananas, peaches, pears, strawberries, and blueberries are among the fruits available.

Grains include whole grain bread, whole grain pasta, quinoa, brown rice, and oats.

Lentils, chickpeas, black beans, and kidney beans are examples of legumes.

Almonds, walnuts, cashews, pistachios, and macadamia nuts are examples of nuts.

Seeds include sunflower seeds, pumpkin seeds, chia seeds, and hemp seeds.

Seasonings: salt, pepper, turmeric, cinnamon, cayenne pepper, and oregano

Salmon, sardines, mackerel, trout, shrimp, and mussels are examples of seafood.

Greek yogurt, yogurt, and milk are examples of dairy products.

Poultry includes chicken, duck, and turkey.

Chicken, quail, and duck eggs are available.

Extra virgin olive oil, avocados, olives, and avocado oil are all good sources of healthy fats.

Though there is no one-size-fits-all Mediterranean diet, it is usually high in healthful plant foods and low in animal foods, with a concentration on fish and shellfish.

It has been linked to a variety of health advantages, including helping to regulate blood sugar levels, increase heart health, and improve cognitive function, among others.

The best part is that you can customize the Mediterranean diet to suit your needs. If you don't care for salmon or sardines but like whole wheat pasta and olive oil, start putting together great Mediterranean-inspired meals using things you enjoy.

Chapter 8: COMMON MISTAKES AND HOW TO OVERCOME DOWN MOMENTS

Are you excited to start your intermittent fasting journey? Intermittent fasting could be precisely what the doctor prescribed to help you reduce weight and decrease extra body fat. However, before you jump in, you need to learn how to approach a time-restricted diet. Several intermittent fasting blunders might not only sabotage your weight reduction attempts but also put you in danger of gaining weight.

As a result, we're providing the seven most frequent intermittent fasting blunders to avoid and intermittent fasting ideas to help you stay motivated and lose weight.

1. When You Pick the Wrong Fasting Strategy

Intermittent fasting enables you to consume all of your daily nutrition in one sitting and then fast for the rest of the day. This meal distribution could seem weird at first, particularly if intermittent fasting differs from your regular eating pattern. You'll replace one of many intermittent fasting regimens with your normal three meals each day when you fast.

The most frequent IF error is picking a fast that is excessively hard or just the incorrect fasting regimen for you. Consider this: if your body is used to eating every two hours, a 24-hour fast would certainly deplete your energy and leave you depressed. Similarly, if your everyday routine keeps you up late at night, starting your fast at 5 p.m. is not good. If you begin your fast early in the evening, you risk staying up later than planned without eating.

Success Advice: Do your homework and pick an intermittent fasting regimen that suits your requirements. The fasting strategy you adopt should fit into your current routine and not exceed how comfortable you are with food restrictions. If you're a newbie, 14:10, which involves fasting for 14 hours and planning your meals in 10 hours, is a good option.

2. When you finish a fast, you eat too much.

It's no secret that finishing your first fast will make you feel tremendously accomplished. This pride, however, should not be used as an excuse to overindulge. After a fast, you'll most likely be hungry. And you could believe that the calories you ate after you broke your fast would compensate for the calories you lost while fasting. If you're feeling this way, it may rationalize your want to binge and undo all of your hard work.

One of the main advantages of intermittent fasting is that it lowers insulin levels and encourages your body to use alternate energy sources to burn fat. When you eat after you've broken your fast, your blood sugar and insulin levels jump quickly, ruining your effort and leaving you with a nagging headache, nausea, and jitteriness.

Success Tips: You'll need a strategy to prevent intermittent fasting blunders like overeating. Prepare a nutritious fruit or veggie-packed dinner that you can eat after your fast is over. When eating, chew your meal thoroughly and pauses to digest and drink water. These techniques will make you feel fuller, allowing you to quit eating before you overeat.

3. You Don't Eat Enough Before Starting a Fast

The eating period leading up to your fast is referred to as your "feasting window" for a reason: you're supposed to eat until you're satisfied. The hunger hormone ghrelin urges your brain to eat when you're hungry. When you limit eating, your ghrelin levels rise, intensifying your hunger. During a fast, high amounts of this hormone might make you feel hungry and deplete energy.

Success Tips: Contrary to common perception, if you don't eat enough before your fast, your ghrelin hormone will never be satisfied, and you will feel hungry for the length of your fast. If you want to have a healthy and happy fast, you'll need to feast. As a result, be sure to eat various nutritious foods throughout your feasting window—fruits, vegetables, leafy greens, and lean protein are all excellent choices for satisfying your appetite.

4. You Indulge in Unhealthy Eating During Your Feasting Period

Aside from not eating enough during your feasting window, overeating or consuming unhealthy meals before or after your fast is another typical intermittent fasting error. Though your body benefits the most when fasting, the meals you eat after or before a fast are what will re-energize you for your next fast. So, if you fill up on meals that temporarily raise your blood sugar or make you feel full, you won't get the full advantages of a fast. The success of your fast is mostly determined by what you consume while you're not fasting.

Success Tip: You'll get the nutrients you need to keep your fast going during your feasting window. So, for energy and fiber, eat complex carbs like whole grains, veggies, fruits, and fruits and vegetables. Sugars, starches, and processed meals are all examples of refined carbs. These simple carbohydrates raise your blood sugar and induce a surge of insulin, which your body uses for fuel rather than metabolizing fat. Find the proper dietary guide to help you stay energized, feel less hungry, and lose weight more quickly.

5. You Are Not Consuming Enough Water

Did you know that about 70% of your body is water? To keep hydrated with such a high water content, you'll need to drink many glasses of water. However, the H2O you drink does not account for all of your water intakes. The food you consume accounts for around 20 to 30% of your daily water consumption. As a result, when fasting, you must increase your water intake to compensate for the water lost from your food.

Another typical intermittent fasting blunder is to consume coffee or caffeinated tea first thing in the morning instead of water. Just from the humidity in your breath, you lost roughly a liter of water while sleeping. Caffeinated beverages have a diuretic effect, making you want to pee more often and dehydrating your body. Furthermore, a large quantity of caffeine can negatively affect blood sugar levels, making you more insulin resistant and more prone to accumulate fat.

Hydrate, hydrate, hydrate. Before consuming any coffee or caffeinated drinks, always start your day with a glass of water. Similarly, strive to drink eight to 10 glasses of water each day.

6. You lead a sedentary lifestyle.

Your lifestyle choices have a big influence on how well you lose weight. Your weight loss is greatly influenced by the foods you consume, the quantity of sleep you receive, and even your stress levels. Similarly, if you don't exercise or stay active throughout your fast, your results could stall. To grow muscle and sculpt your ideal body, intermittent fasting, exercise, and an active lifestyle are important.

Success Tips: Because intermittent fasting is a lifestyle rather than a diet, you must approach it as such. Fill your body with nutritious meals, drink plenty of water, and obtain eight hours of sleep every night. Exercise can help you burn 20% more body fat during intermittent fasting, so try to stay active and get in three to five hours of physical exercise every week.

When your results aren't immediate, you give up.

When you don't experience instant effects from intermittent fasting, you mistake giving up. Realistically, losing weight and shedding stubborn body fat will take time. After your first weight reduction, you'll shed water weight or bloat quickly and lose one to two pounds each week. Don't be disappointed if you don't lose weight soon; studies suggest that it's more likely to return if you lose weight too rapidly.

Tips: Embrace your body at every stage of weight reduction. You won't lose weight overnight, but moderate and consistent weight reduction with intermittent fasting is a healthy and dynamic way to help you lose body fat permanently.

When you're just getting started with intermittent fasting, it's only normal to make a few mistakes. However, if you avoid these frequent intermittent fasting blunders and implement these helpful intermittent fasting recommendations into your daily routine, you can lose weight safely and effectively.

Chapter 9: TIPS TO MAKE IT MORE EFFECTIVE

IF can be done in a variety of ways. The number of fast days and calorie limitations differ across the strategies.

According to research, this type of eating can help you lose weight, improve your health, and live longer. Intermittent fasting advocates believe it is simpler to stick to than typical calorie-controlled diets.

Intermittent fasting is a personal experience for each person, and various approaches suit different individuals.

The science behind the most common varieties of intermittent fasting is discussed in this chapter as recommendations on how to stick to this diet.

Intermittent fasting can be done in seven different ways.

IF can be done in various ways, and different individuals prefer different strategies. Continue reading to learn about seven alternative methods to fast intermittently.

1. Make a 12-hour fast every day.

Intermittent fasting can fit different individuals in various ways.

The diet's guidelines are straightforward. Every day, a person must choose and follow a 12-hour fasting window.

According to some studies, fasting for 10–16 hours causes the body to convert fat storage into energy, releasing ketones into circulation. This should help you lose weight.

This form of intermittent fasting regimen could be a decent choice for novices. This is because the fasting window is rather limited, most of the fasting happens when sleeping, and the individual can eat the same quantity of calories every day.

The most convenient approach to completing the 12-hour fast is to include sleep time in the fasting window.

A person might, for example, fast between the hours of 7 p.m. and 7 a.m. They'd have to complete supper before 7 p.m. and wait until 7 a.m. to have breakfast, but they'd be sleeping for most of the time.

2. Observing a 16-hour fast

The 16:8 technique, often known as the Leangains diet, involves fasting for 16 hours a day and then eating for 8 hours.

Women fast for 14 hours a day, men fast for 16 hours on the 16:8 diet. Those who have tried the 12-hour fast and found it unproductive can benefit from this kind of intermittent fasting.

People who fast this way generally complete their evening meal by 8 p.m., skip breakfast the following day, and don't eat again until midday.

Even though mice ate the same total amount of calories as mice that ate whenever they wanted, research on mice revealed that restricting the feeding window to 8 hours protected them against obesity, inflammation, diabetes, and liver disease.

3. Observing a two-day fast once a week

The 5:2 diet requires people to consume a normal quantity of healthy food for five days and then cut their calorie consumption for the remaining two days.

Women typically ingest 500 calories and men ingest 600 calories during the two fasting days.

Fasting days are usually separated over the week. They can, for example, fast on Mondays and Thursdays and eat regularly for the rest of the week. Between fasting days, there should be at least one non-fasting day.

The 5:2 diet, often known as the Fast diet, has received little investigation. In a research of 107 overweight or obese women, it was shown that calorie restriction twice weekly, and continuous calorie restriction both resulted in equivalent weight reduction.

According to the research, the diet also decreased insulin levels and enhanced insulin sensitivity in the subjects.

A small-scale investigation

The effects of this fasting strategy on 23 overweight women were studied. The ladies dropped 4.8 percent of their overall weight and 8.0 percent of their total body fat in one menstrual cycle. After 5 days of regular eating, most of the women's measures reverted to normal.

4. Fasting on alternate days

The alternate-day fasting strategy, which entails fasting every other day, has various versions.

Some people do alternate-day fasting by completely eliminating solid foods on fasting days, while others allow up to 500 calories. People choose to eat as much as they want on feeding days.

According to one research

Alternate-day fasting is good for weight reduction and heart health in healthy and overweight individuals. Over the course of 12 weeks, the 32 individuals dropped an average of 5.2 kilograms (kg), or slightly over 11 pounds (lb).

Alternate-day fasting is a more intense type of intermittent fasting that may not be appropriate for novices or people with specific medical issues. This form of fasting could also be difficult to sustain over time.

5. A 24-hour fast once a week

Teas and calorie-free liquids are allowed on a 24-hour diet.

The Eat-Stop-Eat diet entails going without food for 24 hours for one or two days a week. Many individuals fast from one meal to the next or from one meal to another.

People on this diet plan can consume water, tea, and other calorie-free beverages during fasting time.

On non-fasting days, people should resume their usual eating habits. This way of eating lowers a person's overall calorie consumption while leaving the individual's food choices unrestricted.

Fasting for 24 hours can be difficult, leading to weariness, headaches, and irritation. As the body adapts to this new eating pattern, many individuals find that these symptoms become less severe over time.

Before attempting the 24-hour fast, patients can benefit from a 12-hour or 16-hour fast.

6. Meal skipping

Beginners can benefit from this flexible approach to IF. It entails missing meals on occasion.

People might skip meals dependent on how hungry they are or how much time they have. Nonetheless, it is important to eat nutritious meals at each meal.

Individuals who monitor and react to their bodies' hunger cues are more likely to succeed at meal skipping. People who follow this method of intermittent fasting eat when they are hungry and skip meals when they aren't.

This could feel more natural for some individuals than the other fasting strategies.

The Warrior Diet

The Warrior Diet is a kind of intermittent fasting that is rather intense.

During a 20-hour fasting window, the Warrior Diet entails eating very little, generally only a few portions of raw fruit and vegetables, and then eating one huge meal at night. In most cases, the dining window is just 4 hours long.

This kind of intermittent fasting could be appropriate for persons who have previously tried other types of intermittent fasting.

The Warrior Diet advocates argue that humans are natural nocturnal eaters and that eating at night helps the body obtain nutrients according to its circadian cycles.

People should eat lots of veggies, proteins, and healthy fats throughout the 4-hour meal period. Carbohydrates should also be included.

While consuming certain things throughout the fasting period is feasible, adhering to the rigorous limits on when and what to eat in the long run might be difficult. Furthermore, some individuals find it difficult to consume such a huge lunch close to night.

There's also a chance that folks following this diet won't get adequate nutrients like fiber. This may raise cancer risk and have a negative impact on digestive and immunological systems.

Tips for Maintaining Intermittent Fasting

Intermittent fasting could be made simpler with yoga and mild exercise.

Maintaining an intermittent fasting regimen might be difficult.

The following suggestions can help individuals remain on track and get the most out of intermittent fasting:

Keep yourself moisturized. Throughout the day, drink plenty of water and calorie-free beverages like herbal teas.

Avoiding food compulsions. On fasting days, plan lots of diversions to keep you from thinking about eating, such as catching up on schoolwork or seeing a movie.

Resting and unwinding On fasting days, avoid vigorous activity, while mild exercise such as yoga could be good.

Every calorie is counted. Choose nutrient-dense meals high in protein, fiber, and healthy fats if the selected plan permits some calories during fasting times. Beans, lentils, eggs, salmon, almonds, and avocado are a few examples.

Consumption of high-volume foods. Choose meals that are both full and low in calories, such as popcorn, fresh vegetables, and fruits with high water content, such as grapes and melon.

Increasing flavor without adding calories. Garlic, herbs, spices, or vinegar can be used liberally to season foods. These meals are very low in calories but high in taste, which could help to alleviate hunger pangs.

After the fasting phase, choose nutrient-dense meals. Consuming meals abundant in fiber, vitamins, minerals, and other nutrients helps maintain blood sugar levels and avoid nutritional shortages. A well-balanced diet can help you lose weight and improve your overall health.

Intermittent fasting can be done in various ways, and no one method will work for everyone. Individuals will get the greatest results if they experiment with several styles to find which one best fits their lifestyle and tastes.

Fasting for long periods when the body is unprepared, regardless of the form of intermittent fasting, might be harmful.

These diets might not even be appropriate for everyone. These tactics can increase a person's negative connection with food if they are prone to disordered eating.

Before undertaking any fasting, anyone with health concerns, such as diabetes should see a doctor.

On non-fasting days, it's critical to consume a healthy, balanced meal for the greatest outcomes. If required, a person might seek expert assistance to customize an intermittent fasting diet and prevent difficulties.

Chapter 10: STARTING INTERMITTENT FASTING (HOW TO PLAN IT)

A recent scientific assessment published in the Annual Review of Nutrition looked at 25 trials on intermittent fasting and found that persons who followed this eating regimen lost anywhere from 1% to 8% of their baseline weight. Intermittent fasting can improve numerous metabolic health indicators, such as blood pressure and cholesterol levels. The weight reduction that comes with it—especially when combined with a regular exercise regimen—can lower your risk of weight-related disorders. In general, intermittent fasting has a lot of benefits.

Of course, intermittent fasting comes in various forms, and the one you pick is ultimately up to you. Time-restricted eating is one of the most common types. You fast for a particular time throughout the day and have a defined eating "window" with this style. You could, for example, fast for 18 hours and then eat for six. Alternate date fasting, which alternates between a day of fasting (when you strive to restrict yourself to 500 calories or fewer) and a day of eating, and the 5:2 diet, which alternates between two fasting days and five eating days each week, are two more choices.

Regardless of the style of intermittent fasting you pick, this eating plan requires discipline and some previous knowledge before going in head first. That's why we spoke to a few vets who practice intermittent fasting. They provided their advice on getting started on the diet and staying on track, so you can have the greatest chance of succeeding with it.

Before beginning IF, see a healthcare practitioner if you are pregnant, have a chronic illness, are underweight, or believe you have an unhealthy connection with food.

1. "Begin slowly."

Since February 2020, Lori G., 46, has been intermittently fasting. "I've dropped around 40 pounds and have kept it off most," she adds. "Start slowly," she advises newcomers. For example, you can begin with a 12-hour fast and a 12-hour eating window, gradually increasing to a 16:8 schedule (where you fast for 16 hours and have an eight-hour eating window). You can move to a smaller eating window after that if you like. "About four to five months after I began intermittent fasting, I gradually moved to [fewer meals per] day," she adds.

2. "Make use of the Fast Bar."

Since December 2020, Elise B., 59, has been fasting intermittently. She fasts for 16 to 18 hours every day on average. She admits, "I'm generally fairly nice about it." "However, there are instances when I work late or have mornings when I simply can't make it."

Elise will have a Fast Bar on hand when such times arise, a plant-based protein bar that has been carefully created to fool the body into believing it is still fasting. "I know that if I eat a Fast Bar, it will keep my body fasting," Elisa explains. "It provides what your body requires, so you are not distressed or unpleasant, but you still get the advantages of fasting."

3. "Be specific about why you're doing it."

Kira C., a chiropractor, has been intermittent fasting for almost three years. Kira fasts once a week and say she chose intermittent fasting because she knew it would help her gut health.

Kira points out that it might be difficult to keep if you don't have a specific purpose for following the eating plan. "Make sure you know why you're doing it," she advises. "At times, some hours can be taxing, and you might just feel very bad at the time. Allow your "big why" to motivate you to persevere in the face of adversity. That meant boosting my gut health for me.

4. "Nap in as late as you can for breakfast."

According to Brisco it's simpler to fast overnight and then push out your breakfast hour. "If you normally have breakfast at eight o'clock, consider pushing it until nine or ten o'clock," she advises. "You can then progressively move it to anytime you like, such as 12 or 1 o'clock," Brisco claims that being busy in the morning prevents her from thinking about eating. "I forget about meals until I get to the workplace," she admits. "At some point, I'm like, 'Oh! 'I have to eat!' I was shocked at how long I could postpone my first meal."

5. Drink a lot of water

Strange it may seem, your body can mistake thirst for hunger. One of the reasons why many individuals who practice intermittent fasting advise keeping hydrated is this. "Drinking a lot of water is one suggestion that helped us manage our hunger and stick to our fasting." "Our objective is to drink a gallon a day," says Alexia B., 33, who began intermittent fasting and a "dirty keto" diet with her wife in April 2018. (If you're unfamiliar with dirty keto, it's a more flexible version of the keto diet that permits certain processed foods.)

6. "Find something that fits within your daily routine."

Choosing an eating time that coincides with your frantic workday isn't ideal when obtaining food is difficult even under perfect conditions. As a result, Lori advises you to "find something that fits within your schedule."

"I like spending time with my family over supper. "I usually break my fast at 4:30 p.m.," she explains. She is, however, adaptable when it comes to her fasting. "When there are festivities or lunch with friends, I allow my schedule to be accommodating," she explains.

7. "Don't judge yourself based on what others have accomplished."

Kayla G., a 33-year-old registered dietitian, has been intermittent fasting for over a year and describes herself as a "big admirer" of the eating plan. "Intermittent fasting has allowed me to lose and, more importantly, maintain the last five pounds," she says.

Her fast normally ends between 12 and 1 p.m., and she eats her final meal between 6 and 8 p.m. "My greatest advice is to don't compare yourself to others," she adds. "Find a routine that is most effective for you."

"Don't be afraid to utilize trial and error to find what works best for you and your body," Kayla says, noting that everyone's metabolism and objectives are different.

8. Drink ginger tea

Rachael H., 29, says intermittent fasting has helped her "keep lean muscle mass" and "maintain a healthy weight" for three years. She aspires for an 18:6 schedule, but she gives herself some leeway when she eats.

Rachael adds, "I prefer to seek actual whole foods." She frequently breaks her fast with a fruit and protein smoothie early to mid-afternoon. "I nearly always eat chicken and avocado with various vegetables for supper," she explains. "When I desire anything sweet, I generally eat a protein shake as a snack."

Rachael says she drinks ginger tea to curb her hunger during fasting times. "Drinking ginger tea in the evenings and mornings helps with cravings and keeps me content throughout fasting hours," she adds.

Chapter 11: INTERMITTENT FASTING MYTHS

Ironically, many people have been using IF for a long time.

Nonetheless, some doubters say that this "diet" is for the birds, not to mention ineffectual.

And that's mostly due to the many following misconceptions surrounding it.

Myth 1: The Most Important Meal of the Day Is Breakfast

"Did you hear this a million times in your life?"

It seems you've heard that you should eat as soon as you wake up — or as soon as your stomach growls — this is not the case.

You will lose out on the advantages of extending your fasting time to 14-16 hours (or even longer) each day if you do this.

The objective is to teach your body to utilize fat and ketones as sources of energy.

As a result of this transformation, our bodies maintain muscle mass and function while metabolizing fat.

Plus, you won't even want to have breakfast after a few weeks.

Myth 2: To maintain muscle mass, you must eat often.

"What makes this myth arguably the most ludicrous?"

For starters, you can't be "anabolic" 24 hours a day.

To get the most out of the anabolic stage, you'll need to spend some time in a "catabolic" condition; the idea is to alternate the two and see your fat levels drop while your muscles build.

Sure, if this were a multi-day fast — or a juice cleanse, for example — that would be one thing.

However, when you do IF, you lose less muscle than you burn fat.

The increased release of human growth hormone (HGH) that happens while fasting is one of the reasons behind this.

Muscle development, bone health, and fat reduction are all aided by HGH.

Your body boosts its production during a fast, maybe as a defense mechanism to maintain that valuable muscle intact for the next hunt.

Contrary to ' conventional ' advice imparted to bodybuilders over the previous century, your body does not need to eat regularly to keep your valuable muscle.

We would all wake up with less muscle than we had before going to bed if this were the reality.

When you get up in the morning, you're more likely to notice your abs and have better muscle definition.

In addition, you will feel more alert and invigorated and lose weight.

When we sleep, our bodies go through a natural process of transitioning from glucose to fatty acids and fatty-acid-generated ketones as a source of energy.

Fatty acids are produced from body fat, while ketones created from fatty acids help sustain muscle mass.

In other words, if you practice IF regularly, your body will get more effective at "turning" this metabolic switch.

Myth #3: It Causes Your Metabolism to Slow Down

The good news is that science has shown that this is not the case.

The amount of lean (muscle) mass you have is the key driver of your metabolism, and we've previously discussed how IF leads to a very moderate loss of lean mass compared to fat mass.

On the other side, research has shown that when you reduce your calorie intake regularly, you lose weight, but only around 1/3 of that weight comes from lean (muscle) tissue.

As you might assume, this might contribute to a decreased metabolic rate and weight accumulation over time.

However, there is evidence that adopting an alternate day fasting schedule for only 21 days resulted in a significant increase in the number of fat grams burnt over 24 hours, from 64 grams per day to 101 grams per day.

This is noteworthy and suggests that IF can help with fat metabolism.

"Would you want additional proof?"

Myth #4: It Doesn't Get Rid of Toxins in Your Body

Blasphemy! One of the nicest things about intermittent fasting is how it helps your body become a well-oiled engine by reducing toxic load.

Autophagy, in which your cells remove waste items, is stimulated while fasting.

You are clearing away the "junk" via autophagy when you fast.

This mechanism seems essential for the survival of all of your body's cells and has been linked to a longer lifetime.

The greatest news is that there's even a natural supplement to help you get the most out of your detox, clean your cells, and get the most advantages from intermittent fasting.

It comes in the form of activated charcoal, another fad-turned-lifestyle choice.

If you're new to fasting, it's crucial to use things that help your body's waste disposal process by capturing and escorting toxins.

This is because your body will not be able to manage the toxins discharged into your bloodstream by your body fat when you first begin fasting.

A few products on the market promise to accomplish this, but the one I prefer is Miracoal, which is made from coconut.

Because of its unrivaled capacity to capture and eliminate toxins, this product is one of the few natural medicines that promote whole-body detoxification.

Myth #5: It Isn't Long-Term

So, here's the genuine question you're probably asking yourself right now:

"Are you kidding me? I'm going to eat like this for the rest of my life?"

Of course, it is all up to you, but the fact is that you can.

It should go without saying that the most difficult component of any diet is depriving oneself of urges for an extended period, continually reminding yourself:

"Don't eat that spaghetti dish."

"Don't eat that cookie,"

"Don't eat that extra pizza slice."

Intermittent fasting obliterates that mindset.

Intermittent fasting is a simple technique to manage your food intake without fighting your hunger.

You won't think about eating during your fasting window until you've become acclimated to the routine.

You can also eat healthy quantities without worrying about dessert during your eating window.

Plus, unlike almost any other diet, intermittent fasting enables you to have a social life.

"Did you have supper late one night?"

Simply shift your dining window the next day.

"Do you have a hankering for breakfast one day?"

Okay, at 3 p.m., you can stop eating.

In other words, it's as adaptable as you want it to be, making it long-term viable.

Because, much like working out, the greatest regimen is one that you will stick to and love.

And, let's face it, no one can maintain a low-carb diet indefinitely.

There is no way to survive without pasta.

Intermittent fasting will boost your health in almost every way.

It fosters a healthy and strong mind and body, and it's much more than simply weight reduction.

Chapter 12: THE EFFECTS OF AUTOPHAGY AFTER THE AGE OF FIFTY

Autophagy can be thought of as your body's natural recycling system. Autophagy, which comes from the Latin phrase "self-eating," is a natural process that includes a cell's superfluous or damaged components being broken down and repurposed as building blocks for cellular repair or producing new cells.

Autophagy is a cellular process that keeps cells healthy. It might happen when you're sleeping or fasting for a brief period, or certain drugs can induce it.

This chapter describes the four processes of autophagy, its advantages, and what happens when it goes wrong.

Function

Autophagy has significant impacts both within and outside of the cell.

Autophagy may aid a cell in the following ways:

• Reduce oxidative stress, which is stress on the body generated by unstable chemicals (free radicals) that could cause cell damage.

• Maintain gene stability

• Improve nutrient-to-energy conversion

• Increase the amount of garbage that is disposed of

Autophagy may aid in the following tasks outside of the cell:

• Reduce inflammation

• Improve the neuroendocrine system's equilibrium, including hormonal chemicals controlling nerve activity.

• Assist the immune system in detecting malignancy.

• Enhance the removal of aged cells

Autophagy is thought to reduce a cell's ability to be broken down into pieces as it ages, contributing to the aging process.

Chronic sickness can result from conditions that alter autophagy's regular functions.

The Process of Autophagy

The fluid within a cell is called cytoplasm. Cytoplasm and organelles—small structures with distinct functions—are recycled during autophagy.

This process maintains homeostasis in your body by eliminating sections of cells that are no longer working properly.

When a cell is starved of nutrition, autophagy is activated. Insulin and glucagon, hormones generated by the pancreas and vital in blood sugar regulation, are involved.

When you eat, your body releases insulin; however, when you fast, your body produces glucagon when your blood sugar drops. Glucagon tells your body to utilize glycogen stored in your liver to raise blood sugar levels.

Autophagy is thought to be suppressed by insulin but activated by glucagon.

Cycles of Autophagy

Sequestration, transport, degradation, and utilization are the four phases in the autophagy process once it is triggered.

Autophagy plays a crucial role in maintaining equilibrium. Any one of them, or all of them, can be employed to suit the body's demands.

Sequestration

Two membranes called phagophores stretch around during this process, ultimately enclosing cytoplasm and organelles that would be broken down later.

This double-membrane creates an autophagosome, which is a kind of organelle.

Typically, the contents of an autophagosome are chosen because they fall within a certain range. On the other hand, autophagosomes can be selective and initiate autophagy only when they connect with certain proteins in the cell.

Transport

A lysosome is a sac-like organelle that houses enzymes and proteins that cause biological processes. These could be employed throughout the dismantling procedure.

Because autophagosomes cannot link directly to lysosomes, they must use an endosome as a bridge. An amphisome is an outcome, and it can easily combine with a lysosome.

Degradation

After this fusion happens, deterioration might commence.

The lysosome releases hydrolase enzymes when it connects to the amphisome. The hydrolases break down the components in the autophagosome's initial state.

An autolysosome or an autophagolysosome is a structure filled with broken-down cellular material (amino acids).

Utilization

The amino acids can be reused after being exported from the autolysosome and into the cellular fluid.

This stage is eventually linked to cellular nutritional deficiency.

Amino acids need broken-down products for gluconeogenesis, a process in which the body produces glucose, or sugar, from non-carbohydrate sources.

The amino acids are used as an energy source in the tricarboxylic acid (TCA) cycle, which recycles them to create new proteins.

Types

This chapter has focused on macroautophagy, which is the most common kind of autophagy. Autophagy and macroautophagy are terminologies that can be used interchangeably.

However, there are two other types:

• Microautophagy is comparable to macroautophagy but does not include the usage of a phagophore. Instead, the lysosome sucks the cell's contents so that it can break them down into amino acids and reuse them.

• Chaperone-mediated autophagy is a more precise means of identifying and degrading proteins. Chaperone proteins attach to other proteins to help them fold, a biological process that transforms them into a three-dimensional structure that allows them to function correctly. As their name implies, Chaperone proteins gather these other proteins and assist in their transmission across the lysosome membrane, where they can be digested into amino acids and reused.

Significance

Autophagy could provide several health advantages. As a result, there has been a lot of study on how to activate this mechanism.

Finding techniques to increase autophagy to aid with neurodegenerative illnesses, which harm cells and nervous system connections and suppress autophagy in cancer patients, is of special interest.

Many individuals are interested in modifying autophagy because of autophagy's possible anti-aging qualities and enhanced metabolic impact (namely, the breakdown and use of food as energy).

Drugs for Neurodegenerative Disease

The use of autophagy to cure illness could have a bright future. Researchers are attempting to figure out how to use medications to specifically switch autophagy on or off.

Autophagy malfunction is linked to several neurodegenerative diseases, such as Parkinson's.

Drugs are being tested to determine if they can activate autophagy in persons suffering from the following ailments:

Huntington's disease is a neurological disorder that affects people of all ages.

Alzheimer's disease is a kind of dementia.

• Parkinson's ailment

• Amyotrophic lateral sclerosis (ALS) is a kind of amyotrophic lateral s (ALS)

• Cancer Therapy

Cancer is also linked to aberrant autophagy, although not due to genetics.

Autophagy provides cell-protective features that help to avoid the development of malignancies. Once a tumor has formed, autophagy is thought to keep it from being killed by the usual cancer-fighting systems in your body.

The lysosome element of the autophagy process is being studied as a target for cancer therapy.

Fasting

Autophagy can be induced by going without meals for short periods or longer periods.

This is accomplished by decreasing cellular nutrition. Autophagy is then activated, resulting in the production of amino acids that could be utilized as an energy source to keep the cell functioning.

Because most fasting research is restricted to animal studies, it's still unknown if fasting for longer or shorter periods is beneficial or detrimental to people. It's also unclear if it can be utilized to help people live longer lives or prevent or cure certain diseases.

Fasting, for example, could be beneficial as a supplement to cancer therapies such as chemotherapy to preserve normal cells and maybe improve their effectiveness, according to animal research. However, further research is required to establish whether these findings apply to people.

According to early studies, short-term fasting during chemotherapy treatment is generally safe for individuals; however, it is difficult.

In addition to fasting, low-carbohydrate diets deprive the body of sugars that are simple to get. Because carbohydrates are not readily accessible, autophagy can be initiated to contribute to amino acid production, which may subsequently be utilized to supply energy through gluconeogenesis and the TCA cycle.

Associated Symptoms

The first autophagy-related genes (ATG) were discovered in the 1990s.

ATGs have been connected to various illnesses since then, including neurodegenerative conditions.

The following are some of the diseases associated with aberrant autophagy function:

• Static encephalopathy of childhood with adult neurodegeneration (SENDA): This neurodegenerative condition causes a buildup of iron in the brain, developmental delays in children, and severe impairment in adults. The SENDA gene affects the development of autophagosomes.

• Vici syndrome: A recessive gene causes this progressive neurological illness. For a kid to be impacted, both parents must pass it on. The linked gene influences the maturation and degradation of autophagosomes.

• Hereditary spastic paraparesis (also known as hereditary spastic paraplegia) is a neurological illness that affects the lower limbs and is caused by a recessive gene. While the function of autophagy is unknown, the linked gene prevents the production of autophagosomes and the fusion of autophagosomes with lysosomes.

• Parkinson's disease is a neurological ailment that affects people uniquely. In this scenario, the linked gene is thought to trigger autophagy to selectively degrade mitochondria (a cellular component involved in energy production). Mitophagy is the term for this process.

• Crohn's disease is an inflammatory bowel illness that affects the intestines. When it comes to Crohn's disease, multiple genes have been linked to autophagy. However, these same genes are linked to a variety of different functions. It's uncertain if Crohn's disease is an autophagy-related condition or whether autophagy-targeted medicines might help.

The first neurodegenerative illness linked to autophagy failure was SENDA. This was crucial in determining autophagy's function in treating different neurological diseases.

It's currently unclear how autophagy malfunction affects the buildup of brain iron in people with SENDA.

Autophagy is a crucial mechanism that maintains your body's cells in good working order by recycling old or damaged components. Amino acids are created from recycled portions, which can be utilized as fuel or to make new proteins.

Autophagy dysfunction is associated with some neurodegenerative illnesses that impair the nervous system and its connections on a genetic level.

Autophagy can aid in cancer prevention. However, in rare circumstances, after a malignant tumor has established itself, this could protect cancer cells.

Researchers are investigating how medications and lifestyle changes, such as fasting, could be utilized as supportive therapies for autophagy.

Chapter 13: HOW EFFECTIVE ARE ANTI-AGING DIETS? HERE'S WHAT SCIENCE TELLS US

Many anti-aging diets are advertised as strategies to lengthen your life expectancy.

However, most anti-aging diet research has been conducted on animals rather than people.

Researchers warn that there is a scarcity of research on the health advantages of these diets.

Before starting any new diet, check with your doctor to ensure it's a good fit for you.

For years, various meals, ranging from basic vegetables and "healthy" fats to powders produced from exotic plants, have been touted as the key to a long and healthy life.

However, many anti-aging diets concentrate on reducing your total food consumption or confining your meals to certain days or times of the day rather than on what you should consume.

Calorie restriction, intermittent fasting, fasting-mimicking diets, the keto diet, and time-restricted eating are all examples of these regimens.

All of these things are meant to help you live longer and live longer in excellent health, which is referred to as lifespan and healthspan, respectively.

Much of the anti-aging diet research has been done on non-human creatures, such as bacteria, worms, and rats.

One explanation for this is that since these species' lives are so brief, it's simpler to track them throughout their lives.

People's research also reveals that certain eating habits can help them live longer and age gracefully.

However, other academics warn that research on the health advantages of these diets for humans is limited, particularly when determining whether or not eating a specific manner will help people live longer.

"Despite their recent popularity, there is no compelling evidence that any of the anti-aging diets examined in laboratory animals provide considerable long-term health advantages in non-obese people," Matt Kaeberlein, Ph.D., and colleagues stated in a study published in Science.

In rodents, calorie restriction is beneficial.

Kaeberlein and his colleagues analyzed current evidence on anti-aging diets in the Science study, concentrating on rodent studies and, where feasible, human trials.

Calorie restriction was the most effective anti-aging diet in mouse tests.

This includes the "traditional" calorie restriction diet, in which daily calories are cut by 20 to 50%, and a version in which total calories are lowered, but protein consumption is maintained.

This is consistent with previous studies that look at the other end of the spectrum — the effect of increased food consumption.

Rodents and non-human primates lose life expectancy when they eat more calories than their bodies utilize, according to Michael J. Forster, Ph.D., a geriatric researcher at the University of North Texas Health Science Center.

According to him, the magnitude of this lifetime shortening is determined by how much and for how extra long food is consumed.

"Based on rodent research, one might claim that the difference in life expectancy [between animals] owing to calorie consumption is up to 50%," Forster added.

In which mice fasted for one day between feedings, Intermittent fasting was another diet that Kaeberlein and his colleagues found promising.

However, since mice consume fewer calories overall due to the fasting days, this is also considered a calorie restriction.

Other diets have been researched, but calorie restriction seems to have the greatest influence on the longevity of rats and other non-human creatures so far.

"There is no evidence that any dietary approach other than [calorie restriction] will have a major and widespread impact on health and lifespan," Forster said.

It shouldn't be difficult to eat more healthily. We'll give you our dietary and weight-loss recommendations based on scientific data.

Certain diets help to enhance health indicators.

Despite encouraging findings in rats, Kaeberlein and colleagues concluded that no anti-aging diets are helpful in humans.

"However, there is some evidence in people that [calorie restriction] and comparable diets have anti-aging benefits," they noted.

According to Valter Longo, PhD, a researcher at the University of Southern California Leonard Davis School of Gerontology who researches aging, part of the difficulty with this study is that academics, scientists, and doctors generally operate in solitude.

"What's lacking," he remarked, "is a multidisciplinary approach." "When all [the data] is taken into account, a different picture emerges, with particular dietary treatments consistently linked to health and lifespan."

Because it's difficult to track individuals for decades, most anti-aging diet research focuses on the short-term effects.

Caloric restriction, for example, has been shown to enhance insulin sensitivity and cardiovascular disease risk variables over two years.

Body mass index (BMI), blood glucose levels, blood pressure, and other health indicators have all improved with the fasting-like diet.

While most anti-aging diet research focuses on extending the frontiers of longevity and healthspan, Forster believes researchers should pay more attention to why certain individuals lose physical and mental function as they age.

"What processes and avoidable events contribute to our inability to reach optimum health as we age, making us susceptible to disease?" he wondered.

For the most part, anti-aging diets are safe.

While the further study on these diets is required, "from one standpoint, we already have tremendous knowledge," according to Forster. "Staying at a healthy weight throughout one's life has improved health and lifespan."

Longo also believes that scientists now have enough evidence on the advantages of less severe diets to promote them to certain populations.

While he does not believe that individuals should fast for 16 hours every day for the rest of their life, he does believe that a shorter fast during the day is safe for most people.

"I've never seen any research that shows that fasting for 12 hours and then fasting for 12 hours every day is hazardous," he added.

Additional qualifiers for other diets, such as the fasting-mimicking diet that Longo investigates. But not so numerous that Longo couldn't recite them in under a minute.

Some of his cautions include avoiding performing these diets too often or too severely — or when a person's diet must be restricted for medical reasons.

"What if you limit yourself excessively or for an extended period?" What if you limit yourself at the age of 85? "Well, that could be a major issue," Longo added.

Cold sensitivity, diminished sex desire, poor sleep, persistent weariness, and muscular weakness are possible side effects of severe calorie restriction.

Longo and his colleagues discovered that although a low-protein diet was helpful for persons aged 50 to 65, those aged 65 and over had a greater chance of dying on this diet.

Other studies have linked intermittent fasting, and other restrictive diets have been linked to disordered eating by other studies.

While not everyone who limits their meals to every other day or within an 8-hour window develops an eating problem, certain individuals are at a greater risk.

Longo believes that many individuals would benefit from a fasting-like diet two or three times a year, but not more often.

Other dietary patterns, he noted, that aren't tied to calorie restriction are proven to be advantageous.

This involves eating a low-protein diet (but not too low, particularly if you are an older adult), eating a more plant-based diet, and ensuring that you receive all of the macronutrients you need, notably amino acids if you're vegan.

"While there is a need for personalization [in diets], there are certain things that will help the vast majority of individuals," Longo added.

Chapter 14: DIETING AFTER 50

At any age, maintaining a healthy weight is a worthy objective. It might be more difficult as you grow older.

You might not be burning as many calories as you were younger, but you can still lose weight.

The weight-loss golden guidelines still apply:

- You should burn more calories than you consume.
- Keep meat and poultry lean by eating more vegetables, fruits, whole grains, fish, legumes, and low-fat or fat-free dairy.
- Sugars and meals with little or no nutritional value should be avoided.
- Fad diets aren't worth it since the outcomes aren't long-lasting.

If you're over 50 and want to reduce weight, there are a few extra things you should do.

1. Maintain your strength

As you become older, you lose muscle mass. Strength training can help to compensate for this. In yoga and Pilates, you can utilize weight machines at the gym, lesser weights held in your hands, or your body weight for resistance. According to Joanna Li, RD, a nutritionist at Foodtrainers in New York, maintaining muscle mass is crucial to burning more calories.

"If you continue to eat the same manner you did when you were 25, you will undoubtedly acquire weight." — RD Joanna Li

2. Increase your protein intake

Because you're in danger of losing muscle mass, incorporate one gram of protein every kilogram (2.2 pounds) of body weight into your diet. "Protein also helps with weight reduction attempts since it keeps you full for longer," Li explains. Wild salmon, whole eggs, organic whey protein powder, and grass-fed beef are among the foods she suggests.

3. Drink plenty of water.

According to Li, as you become older, you may not recognize when you're thirsty as quickly. She recommends drinking 64 ounces of water every day. You may drink it or obtain a portion of it from foods like cucumbers and tomatoes, naturally high in water. Check your pee if you're not sure whether you're getting enough water: it should be light yellow.

4. Get a Leg Up on Your Metabolism

Eat smaller meals and snacks more often, and don't spend more than 3 hours without eating. "Because your metabolism is already sluggish, starving yourself slows it down," Li explains. You might not need as many calories as you did when you were younger. Consult your doctor or a trained nutritionist for further information. "If you eat the same way you did when you were 25, you will acquire weight," Li warns.

Chapter 15: 16/8 INTERMITTENT PLAN FOR 7 DAYS

If you've chosen to give intermittent fasting a try, the 16:8 fasting regimen is usually the easiest. You won't have to count calories on your fasting days as you would on the 5:2 diet. You won't require as much self-control as you would with an OMAD (One Meal A Day) plan. The 16:8 diet is straightforward: you eat a late breakfast or a late supper. That concludes our discussion.

So, if you're interested in giving it a go, here's all you need to know about starting a 16:8 intermittent fasting regimen.

What Is 16:8 Fasting and How Does It Work?

- **Plan for 16-8 intermittent fasting**

16:8 refers to 16 hours of fasting followed by eight hours of eating in 24 hours. So you fast for 16 hours and then eat all of your daily nutrition in eight hours.

Sixteen hours without eating seems like a long time until you realize you'll sleep for seven to eight hours out of the 16. Isn't that bad, right?

So, if the notion of intermittent fasting appeals to you but you are worried about fasting for 16 hours straight, it could be simpler than you think.

Is it necessary for me to skip breakfast?

You might have heard or read that following a 16:8 diet implies skipping breakfast. A 16:8 regimen, on the other hand, is incredibly adaptable – and straightforward – when it comes to intermittent fasting. You have complete control over when your 16-hour fast starts and finishes, so don't skip breakfast if you can't live without it.

Alternatively, you could decide to forgo breakfast. That's OK as well. Whatever makes you feel at ease. Breakfast could be an hour or two later, and supper could be an hour or two sooner. Just make sure you eat within eight hours after breaking your fast. You go without meals for 16 hours straight and only consume calorie-free drinks like water, unsweetened tea, or coffee.

How to Make a 16:8 Fasting Routine

So, which 16:8 fasting regimen will work best for you? Fasting should always include your sleep hours, regardless of when you choose to fast. To figure out what hours are ideal for you, consider the following questions:

- Which meal is most important to me?
- When do I feel the most hungry throughout the day?

If you arrange your fasting time when you are less hungry and less eager to eat, you will be less likely to break your fast or overeat during your eating window.

Choose what time you want your eating window to start and finish once you've determined the most important period of your day for your eating window. Set your dining window from 11 a.m. to 7 p.m. if you plan to miss breakfast or have a late breakfast and an early supper. If you can't start your day without breakfast, you could eat between 9 a.m. and 5 p.m.

Simply choose the optimal start and finish hours for you and stick to them. If you keep to a schedule, you'll feel better and be more inclined to stick to your fasting strategy.

On a 16:8 Intermittent Fasting Plan, What Should You Eat?

There are no limits on what you can and can't consume; IF works with any dietary plan. If you're doing intermittent fasting for health reasons – especially trying to lose weight – being aware of what you're eating within your meal window is critical. The typical American diet, high in ultra-processed foods, will not provide you with the health advantages you need.

Make high-quality nutrition the cornerstone of your approach to get the most out of intermittent fasting. In other words, emphasize unprocessed foods, focusing on veggies, high-quality protein, and healthy fats, and saving processed rubbish for a treat.

Weight Loss with 16:8 Intermittent Fasting

Diets don't work, according to the data. They're not long-term maintainable and aren't very effective for weight reduction. You'll shed a few pounds at first, but studies suggest that these adjustments aren't long-lasting. Intermittent fasting is an excellent option. Because IF is a lifestyle change, it is more long-term than any fad diet that tempts you.

IF has been shown in several studies to be a sustained weight-reduction therapy and a viable alternative if weight loss is your aim. According to a 2018 research, IF can help you lose weight without concentrating on calorie tracking, which is a plus if you don't want to put in the effort.

Other Advantages of an Intermittent Fasting 16:8 Diet

Some of the more general health claims are still up in the air, but there's no doubting that 16:8 fasting has a slew of health advantages, including:

- Improved insulin sensitivity: Increased insulin sensitivity has been linked to weight reduction. However, a new study reveals that IF can improve insulin sensitivity even if you don't lose weight. According to new studies, intermittent fasting may also be a therapy for type 2 diabetes. In a case study published in 2018, IF was shown to help patients cure insulin resistance, maintain appropriate blood sugar levels, and eventually wean off their glucose-regulating drugs. Consult your doctor before starting an IF treatment if you're on diabetic medication.
- Lower blood pressure: About 100 million Americans had hypertension in 2016, defined as a systolic blood pressure of 140mmHg or diastolic blood pressure of 90mmHg or higher. When your blood pressure is excessively high, it might harm your body's tiny blood vessels and negatively influence your health. High blood pressure is linked to

various illnesses, including heart disease, stroke, and renal disease. Fortunately, a new study suggests that IF can help you decrease your blood pressure.

- Improved cardiovascular health: A variety of variables influence your heart health, including your weight, blood pressure, cholesterol levels, and blood sugar levels, to mention a few. Although certain eating patterns, such as the DASH Diet or the Mediterranean Diet, have been linked to better cardiovascular health, there have been no substantial studies tying IF to improved cardiovascular health. IF is linked to better heart health outcomes, such as enhanced insulin sensitivity and cholesterol profiles. According to an April 2020 review in the American Journal of Medicine, IF improves cardiovascular health parameters by reducing oxidative stress, normalizing circadian rhythms, and increasing ketogenesis.
- Reduced risk of type 2 diabetes: Losing weight has a substantial impact on the treatment of type 2 diabetes. Fasting-induced metabolic pathways, such as ketogenesis, have been shown in studies to aid weight reduction. While IF seems to offer promise in treating type 2 diabetes, large, randomized controlled studies are needed to confirm that it is a safe and effective way to manage or treat the illness.
- Improved brain health: Keeping your brain well-nourished is critical for improving your physiological functioning. Intermittent fasting is one way to look after your brain's health. Several studies have shown intermittent fasting to benefit brain health by preserving neurons, boosting autophagy, inducing ketosis, and enhancing neuroplasticity. Ketosis promotes the creation of

neuroprotective proteins, the growth of new cells via autophagy, and the formation of new connections in the brain through increased neuroplasticity. And IF may be able to lift your mood. Consider giving the 16:8 technique of IF a try if you want a healthy mind and a nice mood!

Intermittent fasting could also lower your risk of some cancers, and some animal studies show that it could even help you live longer. Intermittent fasting isn't for everyone, and although the advantages are undeniable, it can also have negative consequences.

Risk of a 16:8 Fasting Schedule

If you're pregnant or nursing, have type 1 diabetes, or have a history of eating problems, you should avoid intermittent fasting. You could also encounter:

- Gaining weight. If you eat too much within your eating window, you can gain weight. Plan your fasting and eating windows carefully, so you don't become too hungry throughout your fast. Keep track of what you're eating and how much you're eating throughout your eating window.
- Hunger. You could feel hungry at first. However, carefully planning your fasting and eating periods might be beneficial. Drink lots of water, find activities to keep oneself occupied, and try meditation.
- I'm chilly. Fasting can make you feel cold, but on the 16:8 regimen, it's less common than on more restricted diets like 5:2 or OMAD. If you're chilly, wrap up; the impact will fade as you get used to your new fasting pattern.

- Dehydration of a mild kind. During your fasting time, consume lots of liquids – just make sure they're non-caloric drinks like unsweetened tea or water.

16:8 Beginner's Advice

The 16:8 technique of intermittent fasting is one of the easier protocols to apply; you can simply customize it to your requirements based on your existing eating habits. You can make it easier by doing the following:

- Set your fasting window around times convenient for you; if breakfast is your favorite meal of the day, eat supper a little earlier than usual.
- It's natural to feel hungry at first since you're accustomed to eating at certain times. Allow your body to acclimatize.
- If you're too hungry, you can try distracting yourself, drinking a glass of water, or meditating.
- Based on your objectives, bulletproof coffee can help you avoid hunger while lowering your insulin levels. On the other hand, bulletproof coffee is not a choice if you're fasting to give your stomach a break since it will break your fast.
- Make sure you drink plenty of water.
- Eat a balanced diet that includes complex carbohydrates, lean proteins, and healthy fats at each meal.
- Pay attention to your body. The 16:8 approach might not even be right for you if you feel lightheaded, sick, faint, or unsteady.

If you're a woman, fasting for more than 12-14 hours can cause you to have an undesirable physiological reaction. Slowly work your way up to a 16:8 fast; start with a 12-hour fast and gradually go to 16.

If you want to explore intermittent fasting, the 16:8 diet might be a good place to start. It's easy and versatile, and you can tailor your eating window to meet your specific requirements.

Chapter 16: INTERMITTENT FASTING AND MENOPAUSE

If you are between 35 and 65, you're probably experiencing symptoms due to the continuous hormone decline. Hormone homeostasis is crucial since hormone receptors can be found throughout our bodies. You can begin to realize that maintaining your typical healthy body weight becomes considerably more difficult as your menopausal hormones change. This might be especially challenging if menopausal desires and appetite are out of control. Sugar cravings can be intense and invasive during menopause. Bioidentical hormone replacement treatment (HRT) can help you rebalance your hormones, and many women have claimed that it eliminates undesirable cravings, which can lead to stress and weight gain. As women reach perimenopause and menopause, they are more prone to accumulate belly fat, particularly deep within the abdomen (visceral fat). Dropping hormone levels cause body fat to be redistributed from the hips, thighs, and back to the belly, resulting in a shift in fat storage. While gaining a few pounds around the waist is natural, gaining more than 5 pounds can be harmful to your health and lead to heart disease, diabetes, and cancer. The good news is that there are effective weight-loss treatments available. When HRT and Intermittent Fasting are combined, they can have a powerful synergistic impact.

The Hormones That Cause Cravings: A Scientific Look

The variety of hormone changes that occur throughout menopause is likely causing you to seek certain foods in greater amounts than usual. When we consume specific meals, our brain is stimulated, resulting in joyful, good sensations. These positive sentiments encourage us to continue eating such meals regularly. Hyper-palatable meals, often known as 'comfort foods,' are the sorts of foods that trigger this 'happy brain.' They are rapid and simple to digest. Sweet, salty, and/or fatty meals are common comfort foods. The majority of individuals consume this sort of cuisine when they are weary and need a 'late-night snack.' You can minimize your intake of these comfort foods by lowering the number of hours you eat for effective weight reduction by reducing the number of hours you eat.

When all of our hormones are in balance, we can sit down and eat a regular meal, and our hunger hormone, leptin, will be produced at the appropriate amounts, signaling to our brain that we are full and should stop eating. The hormone ghrelin is produced from the stomach and alerts our brain that we are hungry again if we haven't eaten in many hours. When estrogen and progesterone levels are low during menopause, it might increase food cravings and reduce contentment after eating. The good news is that you can directly reduce your hunger by regulating your estrogen levels with HRT, which can also suppress hunger by lowering ghrelin levels and improving the efficiency of the appetite-suppressing hormone leptin.

Intermittent Fasting and Menopause

Intermittent fasting (IF) has also been beneficial for weight reduction and weight management in postmenopausal women. IF doesn't limit what you can eat, but it limits when you can consume it.

The decrease in calorie intake and the influence fasting has on insulin levels are two factors that contribute to body fat loss with IF. Because of hormone changes, weariness, reduced lean muscle mass, poor sleep, stress eating, and other issues, HRT + IF can be highly beneficial throughout menopause.

According to recent research, people who were only permitted to eat within a four-hour window ate roughly 650 less calories each day, which could result in a monthly weight reduction of almost 5 pounds.

Hormones and Intermittent Fasting

According to research, intermittent fasting helps lower body weight, lowering fasting glucose, lowering fasting insulin, lowering insulin resistance, lowering leptin levels, and increase metabolism.

Intermittent fasting was shown to effectively reverse Type 2 diabetes and the requirement for insulin treatment in several trials. Intermittent fasting can help you lose weight by lowering your calorie intake and altering your metabolic rate. Sugars (carbohydrates) flowing in the circulation are not broken down for energy; thus, the excess sugar (calories) is stored in fat cells. Your insulin levels drop while you fast, enabling fat cells to release the sugar they've been accumulating and you to utilize it as energy. This is how intermittent fasting promotes fat burning by interacting with your hormones.

Combining HRT with intermittent fasting may help you lose weight by reducing cravings and increasing fat burning. There is no calorie monitoring or food tracking with IF and HRT, and there are no limits on what foods you can or cannot consume.

Before starting a new diet or altering your medicines, always talk to your doctor. If you decide to practice intermittent fasting, bear in mind that the quality of your diet is quite important. It's not a chance to gorge on ultra-processed meals and hope to lose weight.

Using Intermittent fasting with HRT for women in menopause might be an exciting chance to have a beneficial influence. Intermittent fasting is not suitable for everyone, and it is not advised for those who:

- Have a history of eating problems or are prone to them.
- Are suffering from underlying health issues.
- Do you have diabetes or other blood sugar issues?
- Are under the age of eighteen years old.
- Women who are pregnant or in nursing are possible candidates.

Hormone replacement treatment (HRT) paired with intermittent fasting for menopause can provide many benefits to help you accept this time of life as a new beginning. With Winona's menopausal assistance, you can take steps to protect yourself from the health concerns that come with declining hormone levels as you age. Intermittent fasting combined with bioidentical hormone replacement treatment can help regulate hormones and lose weight, particularly belly fat. When a doctor recommends, hormone replacement therapy (HRT) is a safe and biologically natural technique to recover your vitality. HRT can restore correct hormone levels utilizing bio-similar chemicals to those generated by your body.

Chapter 17: HOW TO PERFORM INTERMITTENT FASTING DURING MENOPAUSE

The normal reduction in sex hormones when women reach their 40s and 50s is known as menopause. The ovaries cease releasing estrogen and progesterone during this period, which causes menstruation to halt. When you haven't had your period for 12 months, you've officially achieved menopause. Amenorrhea, or the lack of a period, isn't the sole sign of menopause.

Menopause manifests itself in several ways, including:

• Dryness in the vaginal area

• Reduced libido

• Anxiety

• Depression

• An increased risk of heart disease

• Chills

• Sweats at night

• Mood swings

Menopause also affects metabolism, which many women are unaware of. The metabolism slows down because estrogen and progesterone levels are out of balance during menopause. Many women gain weight as a result of the abrupt hormonal change.

During menopause, you could become less insulin sensitive, which means you have problems absorbing sugar and processed carbohydrates—a metabolic alteration known as insulin resistance. Insulin resistance is often associated with tiredness and sleep disturbances.

Menopause can be a frightening experience. You might feel as if you don't understand your body as well as you once did, and symptoms like abrupt weight increase might make you concerned and unhappy.

The good news is that intermittent fasting is an excellent technique for easing menopausal symptoms. If you're experiencing weight gain, lethargy, and/or insulin resistance due to menopause, it's worth a go.

Will intermittent fasting assist with the symptoms of menopause?

In a word, yeah. Intermittent fasting can assist with a variety of menopausal symptoms, including:

- Gaining weight. Intermittent fasting has been shown to aid fat reduction in studies, and many individuals find it to be an excellent long-term approach for keeping small.

Insulin resistance is a term used to describe a condition in which Fasting improves insulin sensitivity, allowing your body to handle sugar and carbs more efficiently. It could lower your chances of heart attack, diabetes, or other metabolic problems.

- Changes in mental health:s Anxiety, despair, exhaustion, brain fog, mood fluctuations, and psychological stress are all common symptoms of menopause. Fasting has been shown to boost self-esteem, reduce sadness and stress, and promote overall good psychological changes.
- Fog in the head: Fasting protects brain cells from stress, helping them clear out waste materials, repair themselves, and makes them more efficient, according to animal studies. There hasn't been any research on how fasting affects the human brain, yet greater mental clarity is one of the most typical side effects. Although the data for this advantage isn't conclusive, you can try fasting and see if you notice a change.

How to fast intermittently during menopause

Intermittent fasting is a straightforward process. You choose an eating window that works for you, such as 12 p.m. to 8 p.m., and you consume all of your calories. You fast outside your meal window, drinking only water and noncaloric beverages such as coffee or tea. In other words, you're fasting for 16 hours a day and eating for eight hours. This is known as a 16:8 fast, and it is one of the most basic types of intermittent fasting.

Intermittent fasting has the advantage of being adaptable. Many individuals begin with shorter fasts (14:10 fasts, 14 hours fasting, 10 hours eating) and progressively extend their fast time. Some individuals go so far as to just eat one meal every day. You can experiment with various fasting plans to determine what works best for you.

During menopause, should you attempt intermittent fasting?

Weight gain, insulin resistance, and other typical symptoms of menopause can all be managed by intermittent fasting.

Nonetheless, some individuals could be hesitant to undertake intermittent fasting. Intermittent fasting puts your body under modest stress, so if you have adrenal fatigue or a chronic condition, you might just want to avoid it in your routine.

Pay attention to how you feel if you decide to attempt intermittent fasting. If fasting makes you feel excessively anxious, or if you get weak or unwell during fasting, you should either cut your fast short or stop fasting altogether. It's also worth noting that you don't have to fast every day. You can fast every other day or even a couple of times a week if you want to.

Menopause can be difficult, but with the correct food and lifestyle modifications, you can remain fit, happy, and healthy while your hormones fluctuate.

Chapter 18: SIDE EFFECTS OF INTERMITTENT FASTING

Intermittent fasting has been related to a range of health advantages, including:

Intermittent fasting has been related to a range of health advantages, including:

- reduced heart disease

- reduce blood pressure

- increased sensitivity to insulin

- a decrease in oxidative stress indicators

- better regulation of blood sugar

These discoveries have boosted the popularity of intermittent fasting programs such as:

- time-restricted feeding (TRF)

- alternate-day fasting (ADF)

- fasting regularly

Whether you're thinking about attempting intermittent fasting, you're undoubtedly wondering if it has any negative consequences.

The quick answer is that most individuals can safely fast intermittently. Intermittent fasting, however, has been found in studies to have some modest adverse effects. Furthermore, it is not the best option for everyone.

This chapter discusses nine possible negative effects of intermittent fasting.

1. Cravings and hunger

Hunger is one of the most prevalent negative effects of intermittent fasting, which is no surprise.

If you cut your calorie intake or spend lengthy periods without eating, you might feel greater hunger.

112 persons were randomly allocated to an intermittent energy restriction group research. They ate 400 or 600 calories on two nonconsecutive days each week for a year.

These individuals reported feeling more hungry than those who followed a low-calorie diet with constant calorie restriction.

According to studies, hunger is a common symptom individuals feel during the first few days of a fasting program.

In a 2020 research, 1,422 participants took part in fasting regimes that lasted 4–21 days. During the first several days of the regimens, they suffered hunger sensations.

As a result, hunger pangs can fade as your body adjusts to regular fasting intervals.

2. Lightheadedness and headaches

Intermittent fasting is often associated with headaches. They usually happen in the first few days of a fasting regimen.

In a study published in 2020, researchers looked at 18 papers, including persons who practiced intermittent fasting. Some individuals in the four trials who reported adverse effects indicated they experienced minor headaches.

Researchers have discovered that "fasting headaches" are frequently situated in the brain's frontal area, with pain that is mild to moderate in severity.

Furthermore, persons who suffer from headaches often are more likely to suffer from headaches when fasting than those who do not.

Low blood sugar and caffeine withdrawal, according to research, can lead to headaches during intermittent fasting.

3. Problems with digestion

If you undertake intermittent fasting, you can encounter digestive disorders such as constipation, diarrhea, nausea, and bloating.

The decrease in food intake that various intermittent fasting regimes entail may severely impact your digestion, resulting in constipation and other unpleasant side effects. Additionally, dietary modifications connected with intermittent fasting regimens might result in bloating and diarrhea.

Dehydration can exacerbate constipation, another typical adverse effect of intermittent fasting. As a result, it's critical to keep well hydrated when fasting intermittently.

Constipation can be avoided by eating nutrient-dense, fiber-rich meals.

4. Angry moods and other mood swings

When individuals practice intermittent fasting, they can suffer irritation and other mood swings. When your blood sugar levels are low, you could get irritable.

Hypoglycemia, or low blood sugar, can occur during times of calorie restriction or fasting. Irritability, anxiousness, and poor focus are all possible outcomes.

A 2016 research of 52 women revealed that individuals were considerably more irritable during an 18-hour fasting phase than during a non-fasting time.

Interestingly, the researchers discovered that, although the ladies were irritated towards the conclusion of the fasting period, they also felt a greater feeling of accomplishment, pride, and self-control than they did at the beginning.

5. Tiredness and a lack of energy

According to studies, some persons who practice different forms of intermittent fasting report weariness and poor energy levels.

Intermittent fasting might make you feel tired and weak due to low blood sugar. In addition, intermittent fasting can produce sleep disruptions in certain persons, resulting in fatigue throughout the day.

On the other hand, intermittent fasting has been shown in some studies to decrease tiredness, particularly when your body adapts to regular fasting intervals.

6. Bad odor

Bad breath is an unpleasant side effect that some individuals experience when they fast intermittently. Lack of salivary flow and an increase in acetone in the breath cause this.

Fasting enables your body to burn fat as a source of energy. Because acetone is a waste product of fat metabolism, it accumulates in your blood and breath while you fast.

Dehydration, which is a sign of intermittent fasting, can also produce dry mouth, contributing to foul breath.

7. Sleep deprivation

According to some studies, sleep difficulties, such as inability to fall or remain asleep, are among the most prevalent negative effects of intermittent fasting.

In a 2020 research, 1,422 participants took part in fasting regimes that lasted 4–21 days. According to the research, fasting caused sleep disruptions in 15% of the subjects. This was mentioned more often than other negative effects.

Because your body excretes huge quantities of salt and water via the urine, fatigue is more typical in the early days of an intermittent fasting diet. Dehydration and low salt levels might result as a result of this.

On the other hand, other research has shown that intermittent fasting has no impact on sleep.

Research published in 2021 looked at 31 obese persons who fasted on alternate days while simultaneously eating a low-carb diet for six months. This regimen did not affect sleep quality or duration, or insomnia severity, according to the research.

Similar findings were found in research conducted in 2021.

8. Dehydration

As previously stated, the body discharges a lot of water and salt in the urine during the first few days of fasting. Natural diuresis, or natriuretic of fasting, is the term for this process.

You might get dehydrated if this occurs to you and you don't restore the fluids and electrolytes you lost via pee.

In addition, those who practice intermittent fasting might forget to drink or drink insufficiently. This is particularly true when you start an intermittent fasting program.

Drink water throughout the day and keep an eye on the color of your urine to remain adequately hydrated. It should ideally be the hue of light lemonade. You could be dehydrated if your urine is black.

9. Malnutrition

Intermittent fasting, if done incorrectly, can result in malnutrition.

Malnutrition can occur when a person fasts for lengthy periods and does not refill their body with necessary nutrients. The same can be said for unplanned, long-term energy restriction diets.

On different forms of intermittent fasting regimens, people can often satisfy their calorie and nutritional demands.

However, if you don't properly plan or follow your fasting program over a lengthy period or purposely limit calories to an excessive degree, you risk malnutrition and other health problems.

That's why, while fasting intermittently, it's critical to eat a well-balanced, healthy diet. Make sure you're not restricting your calorie intake too much.

A healthcare expert familiar with intermittent fasting can assist you in developing a safe diet that offers the optimum quantity of calories and nutrients for you.

Who should refrain from fasting regularly?

Intermittent fasting could be a good idea for some individuals, but it isn't suitable or safe for others.

Intermittent fasting has the potential to cause hazardous adverse effects in certain persons.

Healthcare experts often advise against intermittent fasting for the following people:

- women who are pregnant or who are breast-feeding

- children and teenagers in their early years

- those in their eighties and nineties who are feeble

- persons who are immunocompromised

- persons who are now or have previously struggled with eating problems

- Dementia patients

- people who have had a catastrophic brain injury or have suffered from post-concussive syndrome

There are outliers to this list, which is not comprehensive. Fasting, for example, has been used to treat epilepsy in youngsters by medical experts.

If you have a medical condition or are already taking drugs, talk to a trusted healthcare provider about the advantages and dangers of intermittent fasting.

Because some individuals are more susceptible to the negative consequences of fasting, it's crucial to figure out whether intermittent fasting is a good fit for your requirements.

Furthermore, if you encounter long-term adverse effects from intermittent fasting, it might be a clue that it isn't working for you. The following are examples of possible negative effects:

- Severe hunger

- nausea

- irritability

- headaches

- fatigue

- faintness

If you're unhappy with intermittent fasting, don't keep doing it.

Even while fasting has been linked to health advantages, there are many more ways to improve your health that do not include fasting.

Following a well-balanced and healthy diet, getting enough sleep, exercising regularly, and managing stress are essential for overall health.

Intermittent fasting has been related to various health advantages, including reduced heart disease risk factors, weight reduction, better blood sugar management, and more.

Intermittent fasting is usually safe, although studies have shown that it can cause hunger, constipation, irritability, headaches, and poor breath.

In addition, several healthcare specialists advise against intermittent fasting. People who are pregnant, breastfeeding, or chestfeeding and those who have eating issues fall under this category.

If you're thinking about attempting intermittent fasting, talk to your doctor first to be sure it's a safe and healthy option for you.

Chapter 19: HOW TO INTEGRATE FASTING INTO YOUR EVERYDAY LIFE

Fasting can be done in various ways, so it is something that everyone can include in their lives in some manner. With that in mind, it's critical to select a fasting regimen that works for you. There is no right or wrong method to fast; the suitable one for you will blend into your lifestyle, encourage an efficient day, and feel long-lasting.

This chapter will cover some considerations to keep in mind while picking a fasting plan that is right for you. After you've evaluated everything, you can start tailoring a fasting regimen to your specific demands and lifestyle.

When are you busiest, and what is your work routine like?

Plan your fasts around your schedule – fast when you're pressed for time and eat when you have more time to prepare and digest. Fasting in the morning is ideal for most individuals since it is the busiest day.

Skipping a meal or two will save you time, but it will also boost your productivity. Fasting increases clarity and attention, which will help you get through your to-do list faster. Fasting will also be made simpler if you have a hectic job schedule. Your thoughts will be diverted from eating, which will assist in alleviating hunger.

When do you have dinner with your friends and family?

It is beneficial to one's health to sit down and enjoy a meal with friends and family. Choose a fasting window when you're less likely to eat with others, such as early in the morning when everyone is hurrying out the door or late at night when everyone is occupied with activities.

Keep this part of your day and fast around these times if you normally eat breakfast, lunch, or supper with friends and family. It is sacred to eat and spend time with others.

When do you become the most hungry or eat the most?

Do you have a king's breakfast, a prince's lunch, and a pauper's dinner? Or does the notion of meals make you nauseous in the morning? Follow your gut instincts and your hunger.

Breakfast isn't required, contrary to common opinion. It's normal (and recommended) to have your first meal later in the day if you're not hungry when you get up. Similarly, if your hunger gradually decreases as the day progresses, consider missing your evening meal.

Center your eating window around your appetite when you are most hungry —this will be different for everyone.

When do you work out?

Fasting and exercise are complementary; thus, fasting while exercising is a good idea. Fasting boosts exercise performance and outcomes, whereas exercise increases the advantages of fasting (autophagy, glucose clearance, etc.)

Exercise can also help you stick to your fasting schedule by distracting you from eating and acting as an appetite suppressant.

If you usually work out first thing in the morning, skip breakfast. If you work out in the evening, start and finish eating earlier in the day to work out with a lighter stomach.

What are your objectives and ambitions, and where are you on your road to better health?

Figure out where you are in your health journey and what you want to accomplish. Start gently if you're new to intermittent fasting or haven't yet developed fat tolerance. Reduce your typical eating window by half an hour each day until you reach a time frame that is comfortable for you.

A 24–72 hour fast, on the other hand, could be beneficial if you need to swiftly lower your blood sugars or reset your appetite. Long fasts are an effective strategy to lower blood sugar and swiftly put the body into ketosis, but they are difficult.

Suppose you're a seasoned intermittent faster trying to break through a fat loss plateau or take your fasting regimen to the next level. Extended fasts on a weekly, monthly, or annual basis can be an intelligent alternative.

Keep in mind that nothing is fixed in stone.

Life is in constant movement, and each day is unique. Similarly, your fasting regimen should be adaptable enough to fit into your routine. Nothing is fixed in stone, and breaking your fast an hour sooner than planned will not affect your outcomes.

Allowing yourself the freedom to fast according to your lifestyle and how you're feeling will almost certainly result in improved adherence. Simply being more aware of hunger signals and keeping track of when you eat and when you don't is a simple and effective method to incorporate fasting into your everyday routine.

Make intermittent fasting a natural extension of your life, rather than following it like a rule book. There's something for everyone, so have fun experimenting and seeing what works best for you.

Chapter 20: FASTING TIPS FOR WOMEN ABOVE 50

1. Things to remember if you're a woman over 50 who wants to try intermittent fasting

One of the most popular diet fads these days is intermittent fasting. Fitness fans and celebrities alike praise this trendy eating-fasting practice for its many health advantages. The alternating eating and fasting dietary pattern is based on the idea that depriving the body of food for a certain period improves the body's efficiency. Furthermore, fasting is a safe strategy that has few long-term adverse effects. However, to get the most out of this eating pattern, women in their 50s must take additional precautions.

2. Why should women over the age of 50 exercise caution while attempting intermittent fasting?

There are various reasons why women over 50 should exercise more caution while attempting Intermittent Fasting than those in their 30s and 20s. To begin with, they have a slower metabolism, and there is a risk that they'd have hormonal disorders, making it harder for them to make a significant adjustment in their diet. They might be somewhat more stressed than others. Women over 50 should adjust their fasting approach to account for these characteristics for better outcomes.

3. Fast for extended periods

Fasting is only beneficial if done properly and for a lengthy period. Fasting for extended periods can help you achieve your health goals more quicker. Fasting for lengthy periods could seem tough at first, but you will get used to it with practice. It's the most effective approach to keeping track of your daily calorie consumption, which is necessary to maintain the shape or remain in shape. Fasting for a shorter period is ineffective.

4. Consume sufficient protein

When following a diet, protein consumption is important for various reasons. It is the cellular building block. Increased protein consumption aids in the replacement of fat cells with lean muscle. Protein also aids in keeping you satiated for extended periods. As a result, if you consume enough protein within your meal window, you can feel less hungry later in the day.

5. Keep yourself hydrated

When fasting, most individuals forget to drink water, which might reduce the advantages of intermittent fasting. When fasting, water aids in the removal of toxins from the body and makes you feel fuller. If you don't drink enough water while fasting, you'll get very dehydrated and in the hospital. So, if you're attempting to lose weight, drink enough water to get the most out of your fasting period.

6. You're not keeping track of your sleep pattern

Poor sleep habits might potentially harm intermittent fasting advantages. You Might have consumed additional calories the day before and increased stress levels. As a result, if you're doing intermittent fasting, optimizing your sleeping pattern might help you get more out of it. Go to bed, wake up on time, and maintain a healthy lifestyle.

Chapter 21: ANTI-AGING FOODS EVERYONE OVER 50 SHOULD EAT

Have you ever thought about the advantages of anti-aging foods?

There are so many positive aspects to growing older. Experience, knowledge, and realizing our true selves are all wonderful blessings. The physical impacts of aging, on the other hand, aren't as pleasant. You know what I'm talking about: thinning hair, wrinkled skin, etc.

WHAT ARE THE BENEFITS OF ANTI-AGING FOODS?

Many of us over 50 ladies are on the lookout for medicines and drugs that could help us reverse the signs of aging. While many vitamins and supplements have their place in your daily routine, putting chemicals like those found in most pharmaceuticals into our systems might do more damage than good.

I am so enthusiastic about the anti-aging foods' transforming abilities. We feel the advantages of these age-defying superfoods from the inside out when we consume them. Instead of merely treating aging symptoms, we're addressing the root cause!

These top ten anti-aging foods are tasty and assist in preventing (and even reverse) aging in a variety of ways...

TOP NINE ANTI-AGING FOODS

9. PAPAYA

If you like anti-aging fruits, then #10 on my list is for you. Papaya is tasty and can help you live a better life as you become older. This is because it includes...

Vitamin C: Most of us are familiar with vitamin C as an immune system booster. This is true, but it also aids in the maintenance of collagen levels. Vitamin C keeps our skin lush, firm, and wrinkle-free in this way.

Potassium: Did you know that potassium aids in moisturizing our skin? Our skin is less prone to dry out, flake, or wrinkle if we keep it moisturized.

Vitamin A: Like vitamin C, vitamin A aids in the production of collagen in our skin. Our skin receives a double dosage of collagen when we eat papaya!

Papain is an enzyme found in papaya fruit and is one of nature's most potent anti-inflammatories. One of the best-kept anti-aging secrets is this enzyme. Papain fights free radical damage, which helps prevent wrinkles and inflammation within the body. Inflammation hastens the aging process and may lead to chronic discomfort, diseases, and poor overall health.

Water: Because papaya has a high proportion of water, it helps to keep you hydrated. When you stay hydrated on the inside, your skin will age more slowly on the surface.

A special recommendation! If you spread papaya on flaky skin or a skin tag a few times a day, it will help... It will vanish shortly.

Papaya is one of my favorite fruits to eat simply for breakfast, a snack, or dessert.

8. BLUEBERRIES

Who doesn't like the delicious taste of blueberries? They are one of my favorite fruits. I've been eating blueberries since I was a child, but I wasn't aware of their incredible anti-aging properties until lately. Because of their antioxidant properties, blueberries aid in the prevention of aging...

Vitamin C: When it comes to collagen formation, vitamin C is a force to be reckoned with. Citrus fruits are often the first thing that comes to mind when thinking about vitamin C. On the other hand, one cup of blueberries supplies 24% of the daily vitamin C requirement.

Antioxidants: Did you know that blueberries have the highest concentration of antioxidants of any fruit or vegetable? Flavonoids make up the majority of the antioxidants found in blueberries. Anthocyanins are, in fact, the most common kind.

Anthocyanins have been shown to protect against free radical damage, combat inflammation, maintain collagen levels, protect blood vessels, enhance brain function and memory, and prevent heart disease. As if that wasn't enough, blueberries' antioxidants help protect DNA from oxidative damage. The loss in our mental and physical health is caused by oxidative DNA damage, a normal component of the aging process. Blueberries slow down the aging process! Even though blueberries are #8 on the list, their anti-aging properties are undeniable.

This anti-aging meal can be consumed in a variety of ways. Blueberries can be used in yogurt, oatmeal, baked goods, smoothies, and various other dishes. What's your preferred method of consumption?

7. POMEGRANATE SEEDS

Pomegranate seeds have gained popularity in the anti-aging field in recent years. Scientists have lately found that they are genuinely an anti-aging superfood, despite having been around for years. This is why:

Vitamin C: Pomegranate seeds contain vitamin C, which helps maintain skin plump, smooth, moisturized, firm, and wrinkle-free.

Ellagic acid is an antioxidant that protects against free radical damage. Free radicals damage our cells, speeding up the aging process.

Punicalagin: Although it's difficult to pronounce, punicalagin is a potent anti-aging substance. Punicalagin is a one-of-a-kind chemical because it boosts collagen formation. Many other compounds aid in stabilizing collagen formation, but this one increases it. Collagen is the protein that keeps our skin looking thick and full.

Antioxidants: Pomegranates, like blueberries, contain an antioxidant called anthocyanins. Anthocyanins perform all of the functions stated above and assist in the prevention of solar damage.

Pomegranate seeds are delicious on their own or in salads, cereals, and yogurt. They're perfect for a mid-afternoon snack!

6. PINEAPPLE

Pineapple isn't often seen on anti-aging food lists. It does, however, have some amazing anti-aging qualities.

Pineapple is high in...

Bromelain: Bromelain is an enzyme that has anti-inflammatory properties. Bromelain is often recommended to minimize edema and redness after surgery. Skin inflammation can make us seem much older than we are.

Manganese stimulates the enzyme prolidase, which aids in the formation of collagen. The quantity of collagen in our skin gradually decreases as we get older, leaving us with thin, drooping skin. Manganese can both prevent and reverse this issue.

Pineapples are made up of 85 percent water. That is to say, they assist you in staying hydrated, which we all know is essential for good skin. Your skin will become less dry and wrinkled as it becomes more moisturized.

Smoothies, yogurt, and fruit salads all benefit from the addition of pineapple. You may eat it on its own as well!

5. SWEET POTATOES

Sweet potatoes are an excellent source of anti-aging nutrients. They've been touted as a healthy meal for a long time with a good cause! They're not only a delicious alternative to starchy white potatoes, but they're also loaded with vitamins and minerals, including...

Beta-carotene can be found in a variety of orange fruits and vegetables. It's high in vitamin A, which helps regulate oil production, even out pigmentation, and boost collagen formation. In a nutshell, vitamin A is undoubtedly one of the most effective anti-aging substances available.

Vitamin C maintains the plumpness and firmness of your skin.

These components, potassium and pantothenic acid, are excellent moisturizers. It's even more crucial to keep our skin hydrated as we get older. The absence of estrogen during menopause can result in dry and oily skin. These illnesses benefit from potassium and pantothenic acid, which are anti-aging substances!

Folate is a nutrient that is suggested for women of all ages. Pregnant women take folate to avoid birth abnormalities. Women over the age of 50 should take folate to aid brain function.

Sweet potatoes are an anti-aging meal that can be cooked, mashed, fried, or combined with other ingredients to make casseroles.

4. WALNUTS

Walnuts are underappreciated. Health publications sometimes label them as "unhealthy" due to their excessive fat content. But it's exactly because of this that they're such a great anti-aging meal! High-fat foods like walnuts are now known to be vital for brain health. They include...

Omega-3 fatty acids: Everyone need a sufficient amount of omega-3 fatty acids in their diet. These fatty acids have been shown to boost brain function, raise good cholesterol levels, decrease inflammation, and promote collagen production. Omega-3 fatty acids, in summary, aid in preventing dementia, keep your body healthy and keep your skin looking young.

Phytochemicals: Polyunsaturated fats are phytochemicals present in walnuts. These substances aid in the prevention of wrinkles and the reduction of the risk of heart disease.

Walnuts are delicious on their own or sprinkled over salads and desserts. This anti-aging meal goes well with something sweet like fruit. Walnuts have a savory taste that pairs well with sweet fruit.

3. CAPSICUM RED (BELL PEPPER)

Red capsicum, sometimes known as bell pepper in the United States, is an underappreciated anti-aging vegetable. It includes two anti-aging super-ingredients that can significantly improve your body's appearance:

Who doesn't desire lush, firm, and robust skin long into their 50s? Vitamin C can help. Vitamin C will provide you with just that.

Carotenoids are a form of antioxidant that helps prevent inflammation and environmental pollutants and slow the aging process and improve eyesight.

You can have the skin of your dreams by using red capsicum in your everyday diet! Plus, better eyesight and a slower aging process never harmed anybody!

2. AVOCADO

Avocado is one of my favorite foods. I adore it so much. It is one of the greatest meals to consume if you want your skin to be hydrated and free of blemishes. It is, nevertheless, a potent anti-aging meal. This is why:

Carotenoids: Lutein is the most common form of the carotenoid present in avocado. Lutein protects against UV skin damage and macular degeneration, which causes vision loss.

Boron is a mineral that has been shown to help with bone density, coordination, and brain function. It's so powerful that athletes often use it to improve their performance.

Chlorophyll: This antioxidant is responsible for the beautiful color of avocados and other green fruits and vegetables. But it does a lot more. Free radical damage is known to be prevented by chlorophyll. The aging process is accelerated by free radical damage. So, if you eat one avocado every day, you will live longer!

Omega-3 fatty acids help to decrease inflammation, enhance cognitive function, and boost collagen formation, among other things. They are one of the most effective anti-aging substances available.

Avocado can be eaten on its own, but I like it on toast, salads, or guacamole. However, by adding this creamy anti-aging food to smoothies and puddings, you may attempt a variety of innovative dishes.

1. BROCCOLI SPROUTS

They are, without a doubt, the finest anti-aging food on the planet. It's all down to a single ingredient: sulforaphane.

Broccoli sprouts contain the highest concentration of sulforaphane of any food.

Many cruciferous vegetables contain the chemical sulforaphane. This miraculous substance can...

- Reduce Inflammation
- Boost your brainpower
- Prevent Cancer
- Reduce your blood pressure.
- Reduce your chances of developing heart disease.
- Heart attacks can be avoided.
- Toxic substances in the environment should be avoided.
- Boost your energy levels

Can you understand why I like broccoli sprouts so much?

Broccoli sprouts are a powerful anti-aging vegetable that I consume daily. In reality, I'm the one who grows them! They are not only good for you, but they're also inexpensive.

There is one thing you should know about broccoli sprouts, however. To get the advantages of sulforaphane, you must chew it! The chemical is released in this manner.

Freeze your broccoli sprouts to boost their nutritional value!

ANTI-AGING FOODS SHOULD BE INCLUDED IN YOUR DIET!

Chapter 22: RECIPES FOR INTERMITTENT FASTING

BREAKFAST

1. Trail Mix

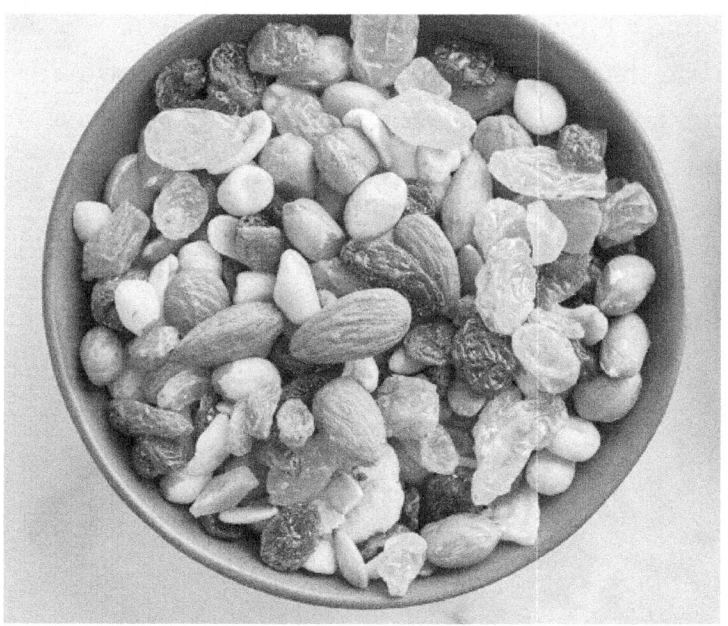

Ready in: 2mins

Serves: 6

Ingredients

- 1 cup sunflower seeds (raw)
- 1 cup almonds (raw)

- 1 cup raisins
- 1/4 cup flaked coconut (optional)
- 1/2 cup dried apricot (unsulphured, chopped)
- 1/4 cup carob chips (optional) or 1/4 cup chocolate (optional)

Directions

1. Pour it all into a big container, cover it and shake it!
2. Store in a bag that is airtight. To preserve the properties of the essential fatty acids, place them in the fridge/freezer.

2. Warm Roasted Vegetable Farro Salad

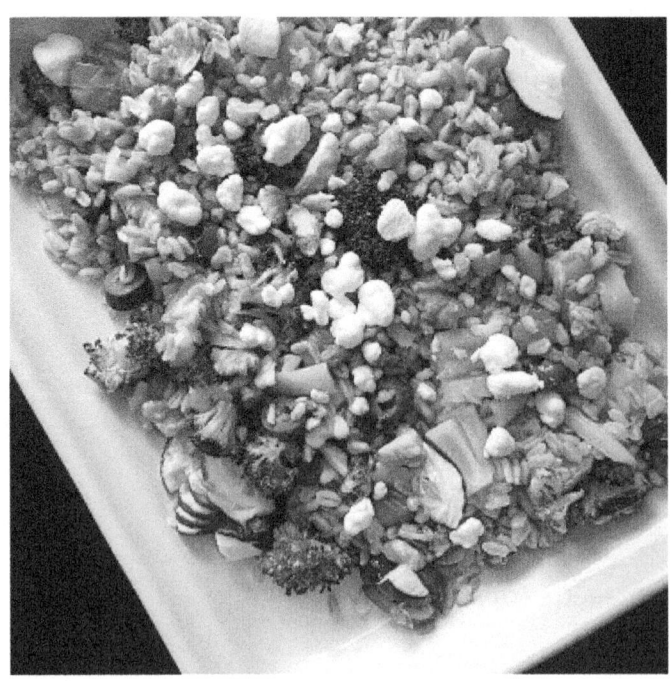

Ready in: 1hr 35mins

Serves: 4

Yield: 4

Ingredients

- One tablespoon kosher salt or One tablespoon sea salt
- 1/2 medium-sized eggplant, peel on, and large diced
- One cup cherry tomatoes washed and left whole
- Six white button mushrooms, quartered
- One medium-sized zucchini, peel on and large diced
- Six garlic cloves, peeled, trimmed, and sliced
- 1/2 medium-sized red onion, peeled and cut into wedges
- 1 cup cracked farro
- 2 cups almond milk (Almond Breeze)
- One tablespoon olive oil
- One teaspoon tbsp olive oil (15 mL)
- One tablespoon balsamic vinegar
- 3 sprigs fresh cilantro
- One tablespoon olive oil
- 1/2 teaspoon salt
- 1/2 teaspoon pepper

Directions

1. Preheat the oven to 200 C (400 °F).
2. Salt the eggplant slices generously on all sides in a wide flat pan or baking sheet, toss to cover evenly, and keep for 30 minutes to release excess moisture and bitterness.

3. Drain the eggplant and rinse and toss it into a large mixing bowl. Tomatoes, zucchini, mushrooms, garlic, and onions are added. Drizzle the vegetables with olive oil generously, season with salt and pepper, and stir to coat. Move the vegetables to a pan lined with ovenproof tin foil. In the oven, roast the vegetables for 20 - 25 minutes or until tender, caramelized, and forked. To avoid sticking to the plate, stir or flip the vegetables about 10 to 15 minutes into the roasting process. Set aside and remove the pan from the oven.

4. Meanwhile, rinse the ferro with water and drain over the sink in a colander. Into a 3-quart (3L) saucepot, add the farro, and add in the Almond Breeze. A pinch of salt and a drizzle of olive oil is added. Bring the liquid to a boil over medium-high heat to prevent boiling, then turn the heat down to a gentle simmer. Simmer the farro with the lid on the pot cocked to one side for 20 minutes to let out steam. Turn off the heat but leave the pot and close the lid on the stovetop. For another 5 minutes or until the farro is soft yet slightly chewy in the middle, steam in the pot. Using a fork to loosen the lid and the fluff.

5. Mix the cooked farro with the vegetables in a large serving dish and gently toss to mix until ready to assemble the dish. Whisk the balsamic vinegar along with the olive oil and drizzle over the farro salad. Toss to coat and season to taste with salt and pepper. Add fresh cilantro and a squeeze of lemon to garnish. Serve it sweet.

3. Cajun Potato, Prawn/Shrimp And Avocado Salad

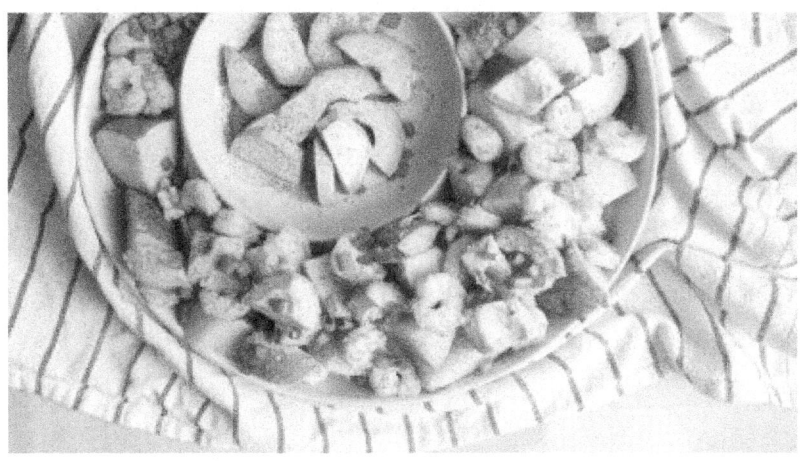

Ready in: 30mins

Serves: 2

Ingredients

- One tablespoon olive oil
- 300 g new potatoes (small baby or chats 10 oz halved)
- 250 g king prawns (8 oz, cooked and peeled)
- Two spring onions (finely sliced)
- One garlic clove (minced)
- Two teaspoons cajun seasoning
- 1 cup alfalfa sprout
- 1avocado (peeled, stoned, and diced)
- salt (to boil potatoes)

Directions

1. Cook the potatoes for 10 to 15 minutes in a large saucepan of lightly salted boiling water, or until tender, then drain well.
2. In a wok or a large nonstick frying pan/skillet, heat the oil.
3. Season with the prawns, garlic, spring onions, and cajun and fry for 2 to 3 minutes or until the prawns are hot.
4. Stir in the potatoes, then cook for an additional minute.
5. Transfer to dishes for serving and top with the avocado and sprouts of alfalfa and eat.

4. Baked Mahi Mahi

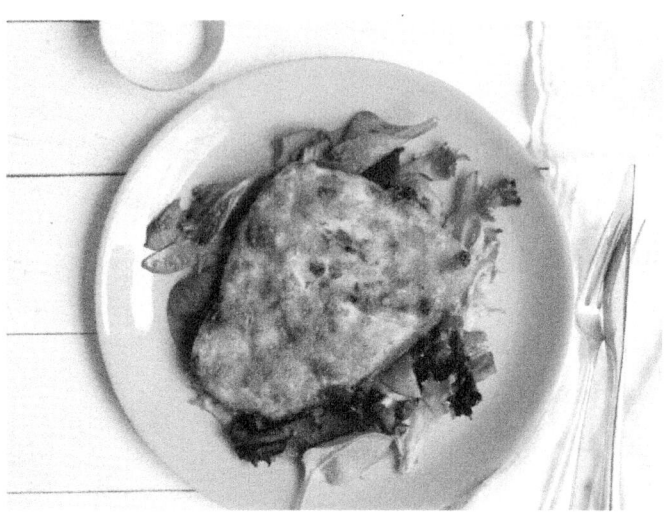

Ready in: 40mins

Serves: 4

Ingredients

- 2 lbs mahi-mahi (4 fillets)
- 1⁄4 teaspoon garlic salt
- One lemon, juiced
- 1 cup mayonnaise
- 1⁄4 cup white onion, finely chopped
- 1⁄4 teaspoon ground black pepper
- breadcrumbs

Directions

1. Preheat the oven to 425 degrees.
2. Put it in a baking dish and rinse the fish. Squeeze the fish with lemon juice and sprinkle with garlic, salt, and pepper.
3. Combine the mayonnaise and the chopped onions and scatter them over the fish. Sprinkle with breadcrumbs and bake for 25 minutes at 425°F.

5. Sheet Pan Chicken And Brussel Sprouts

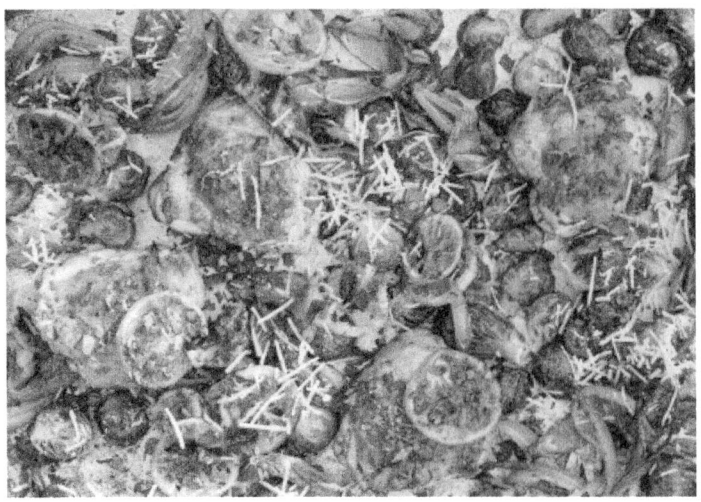

Ready in: 40mins

Serves: 4

Ingredients

- 1 1⁄2 cups Brussels sprouts, halved
- Four skin-on chicken thighs
- Four carrots, cut on the bias
- One teaspoon herbs de Provence
- Three tablespoons olive oil

Directions

1. Preheat the stove to 400o F.
2. Put the cut vegetables in a bowl and add 11⁄2 tablespoons of olive oil, 1⁄2 tablespoons of herbs, salt, and pepper. Rub the vegetables all over.
3. On a sheet pan, place the veggies.

4. In the same bowl, add the chicken thighs. Drizzle with 1½ tablespoons of olive oil, ½ tablespoons of herbs, salt, and pepper. Rub the chicken all over.
5. Put the chicken in a pan.
6. Roast for 30-35 minutes or until you're done with the chicken.
7. Turn the oven over to broil and cook for a minute or two if you prefer a crispier vegetable or chicken skin. Carefully watch, or it'll burn.

6. Perfect Cauliflower Pizza Crust

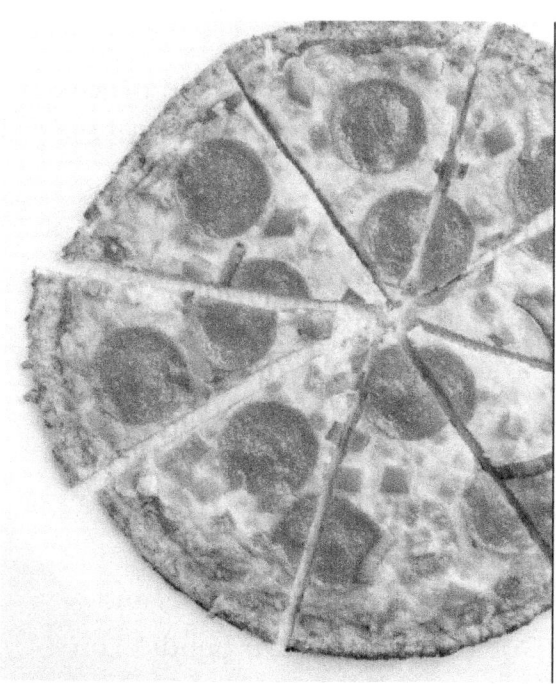

Ready in: 1hr 10mins

Serves: 4

Ingredients

- One egg, beaten
- Four cups raw cauliflower, riced, or one medium cauliflower head
- One cup chevre cheese or 1 cup other soft cheese
- One pinch salt
- One teaspoon dried oregano

Directions

1. Preheat to 400°F in your oven.
2. Pulse batches of raw cauliflower florets in a food processor to render the cauliflower rice until a rice-like texture are achieved.
3. Fill a big pot and bring it to a boil with around an inch of water. Connect the "rice" and cover; cook for 5 minutes or so. Drain the strainer into a fine-mesh one.
4. THIS IS THE SECRET: Move it to a clean, thin dishtowel once you've strained the rice. In the dishtowel, cover the steamed rice, curl it and Suck out all the excess moisture! It's amazing how much extra liquid will be released, leaving you with a good dry crust of the pizza.
5. Mix your strained rice, beaten egg, goat's cheese, and spices in a big bowl. (Don't fear using your hands! You want it mixed well.) It's not going to be like every pizza dough you've ever dealt with, yet don't worry, it's going to stay together!

6. On a baking sheet lined with parchment paper, press the dough out. Keep the dough about 3/8" thick, and make the edges a little higher for a "crust" effect, if you like. (It must be lined with parchment paper, or it will stick.)"
7. Bake at 400 ° F for 35-40 minutes. The crust should be firm and, when done, golden brown.
8. Now's the time to add sauce, cheese, and any other toppings you want to all your favorites. Put the pizza back in the oven for 400F and bake for an additional 5-10 minutes, only until the cheese is hot and bubbly.
9. Cut and quickly serve!

7. Sweet Potato And Black Bean Burrito

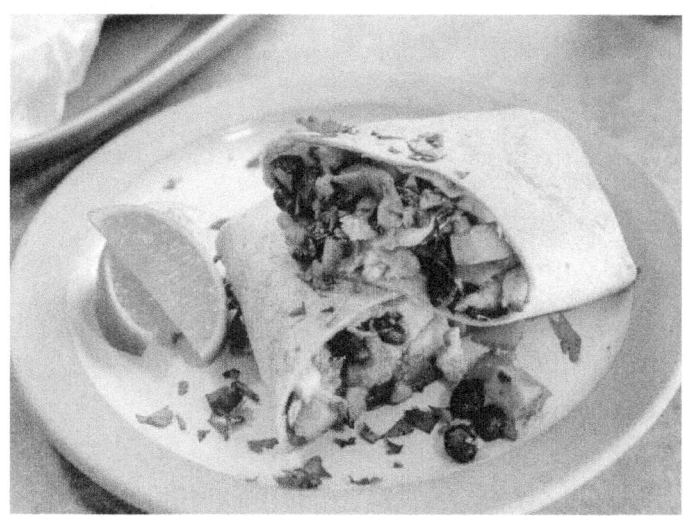

Ready in: 1hr 5mins

Yield: 8-12 portions

Ingredients

- 5 cups peeled cubed sweet potatoes
- two teaspoons other vegetable oil or two teaspoons broth
- 1/2 teaspoon salt
- 3 1/2 cups diced onions
- One tablespoon minced fresh green chili pepper
- 4garlic cloves, minced (or pressed)
- Four teaspoons ground cumin
- 4 1/2 cups cooked black beans (three 15-ounce cans, drained)
- Four teaspoons ground coriander
- 2/3 cup lightly packed cilantro leaf
- One teaspoon salt
- 12 (10 inches) flour tortillas
- Two tablespoons fresh lemon juice
- fresh salsa

Directions

1. preheat the oven To 350*.
2. Place the salt and water in a medium saucepan to cover the sweet potatoes.
3. Cover and bring to a boil, then simmer for about 10 minutes, until tender.
4. Drain yourself and set aside.
5. Heat the oil in a medium saucepan or skillet while the sweet potatoes are frying, and add the onions, garlic, and chili.
6. On medium-low heat, cover and cook, occasionally stirring, until the onions are tender, around 7 minutes.

7. Add cumin and coriander and cook, constantly stirring, for 2 to 3 minutes longer.
8. Remove and set aside from the sun.
9. Combine the black beans, lemon juice, cilantro, salt, and cooked sweet potatoes in a food processor and puree until smooth (or mash the ingredients in a large bowl by hand).
10. In a large mixing bowl, pass the sweet potato mixture and blend in the cooked onions and spices.
11. Oil a large baking dish lightly.
12. At the center of each tortilla, spoon around 2/3 to 3/4 cup of the filling, roll it up, and put it in the baking dish, seam side down.
13. Cover thoroughly with foil and bake for 30 minutes or so, until sweet.
14. Serve with salsa topping.

8. Sweet Potato Curry With Spinach And Chickpeas

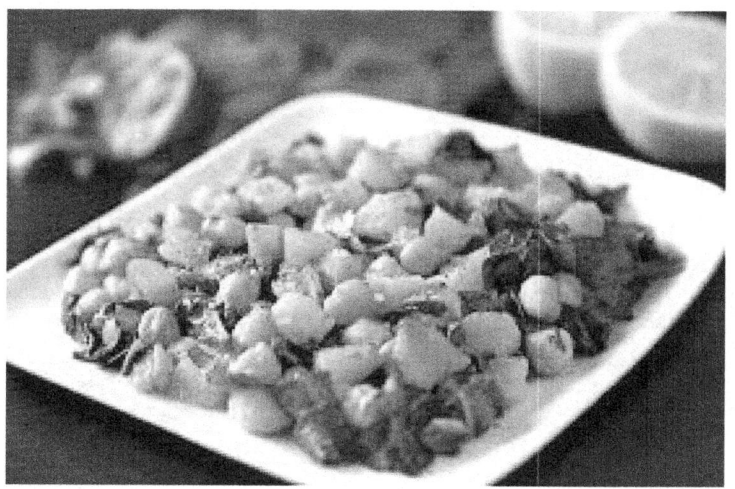

Ready in: 30mins

Serves: 6

Ingredients

- 1 -2 teaspoon canola oil
- One tablespoon cumin
- Two tablespoons curry powder
- One teaspoon cinnamon
- 1/2 large sweet onions, chopped or two scallions, thinly sliced
- ten ounces fresh spinach washed, stemmed, and coarsely chopped
- One (14 1/2 ounce) can chickpeas, rinsed and drained
- Two large sweet potatoes, peeled and diced (about 2 lbs)
- 1/2 cup water
- 1/4 cup chopped fresh cilantro for garnish
- One (14 1/2 ounce) can diced tomatoes, can substitute fresh if available
- basmati rice or brown rice, for serving

Directions

1. Whatever you like, you can choose to cook sweet potatoes.
2. I enjoy peeling, slicing, and steaming mine for about 15 minutes in a veggie steamer.
3. Fit well baking or boiling, too.
4. Heat 1-2 tsp of canola or vegetable oil over medium heat while the sweet potatoes are cooking.
5. Add the onions and sauté for 2-3 minutes, or until tender.

6. Add the curry powder, cumin, and cinnamon, then stir to cover the spices' onions evenly.
7. Stir in the tomatoes and their juices, and stir in the chickpeas to blend.
8. Add half a cup of water and lift the heat for about a minute or two to a high simmer.
9. Then add fresh spinach, stirring to cover with cooking liquid, a few handfuls at a time.
10. Cover and boil until just wilted, about 3 minutes, when all the spinach is added to the pan.
11. Apply to the liquid the cooked sweet potatoes, and stir to coat.
12. Simmer for another 3-5 minutes, or until you mix the flavors well.
13. Move to a dish for serving, toss with fresh cilantro and serve sweet.
14. This dish is served beautifully over basmati or brown rice.

9. Poached Eggs & Avocado Toasts

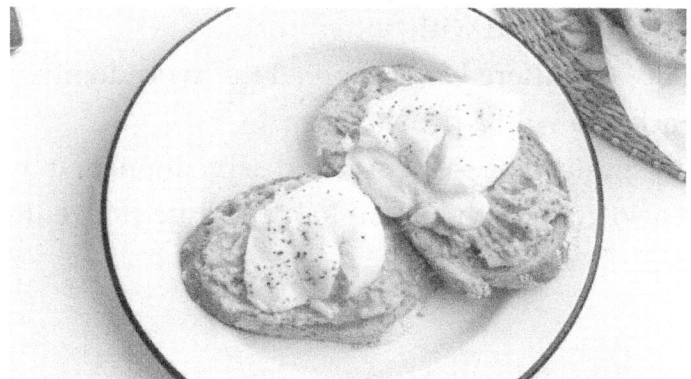

Ready in: 15mins

Serves: 4

Ingredients

- two ripe avocados
- four eggs
- two teaspoons lemon juice (or juice of 1 lime)
- one cup cheese (grated, edam, gruyere, or whatever you have on hand)
- four slices thick bread
- four teaspoons butter (for spreading on toast)
- salt & freshly ground black pepper

Directions

1. Using your favorite technique, poach eggs.
2. Meanwhile, the avocados are cut in half, and the stones are removed.
3. Scoop out the flesh in a bowl with a spoon and apply the lemon or lime juice and salt & pepper.
4. Mash using a fork.
5. Bread toast and spread with butter.
6. On each slice of buttered toast, spread the avocado mix and top each one with a poached egg.
7. Sprinkle the grated cheese over it and serve immediately.
8. These are also good with tomato halves on the side, either fresh or grilled.

10. French Vanilla Almond Granola

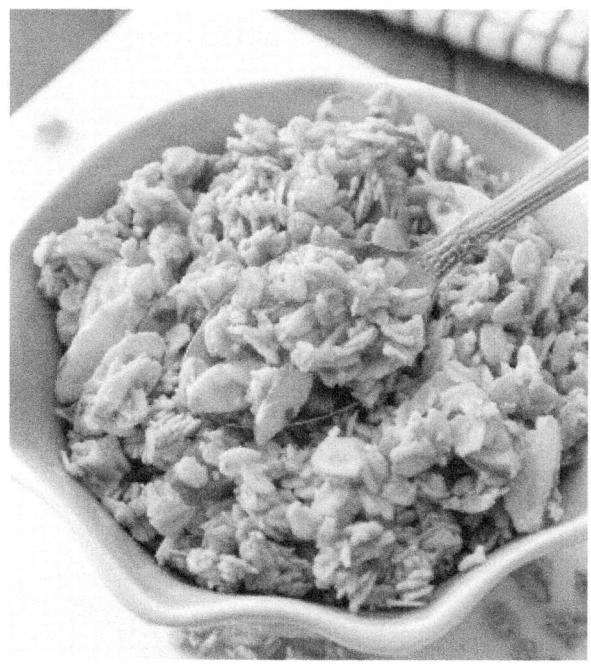

Ready in: 2hrs 10mins

Serves: 12

Yield: 12 1/2 cup servings

Ingredients

- 1/2 cup sliced almonds
- 3 1/2 cups old fashioned oats (not quick)
- 1/2 cup water
- 1/4 teaspoon salt
- 1/2 cup natural cane sugar
- One tablespoon vanilla extract
- 1/4 cup organic canola oil or 1/4 cup grapeseed oil

Directions

1. Heat the oven to 200°F. Use parchment paper to line a big, rimmed cookie sheet.
2. Combine the oats and the almonds in a large dish.
3. Stir the sugar and salt into the water in a small saucepan over medium heat. Stir and cook until the sugar has dissolved. Withdraw from the sun. Stir in the vanilla and canola oil. Pour the oat and almond mixture into the mixture and stir until well mixed.
4. On the lined cookie sheet, spread the mixture out and bake for 2 hours, or until tender to the touch. Oh, don't stir! Remove from the oven and allow to cool into chunks before breaking apart. Store in a bag that is air-tight.

11. Vegan Fried 'Fish' Tacos

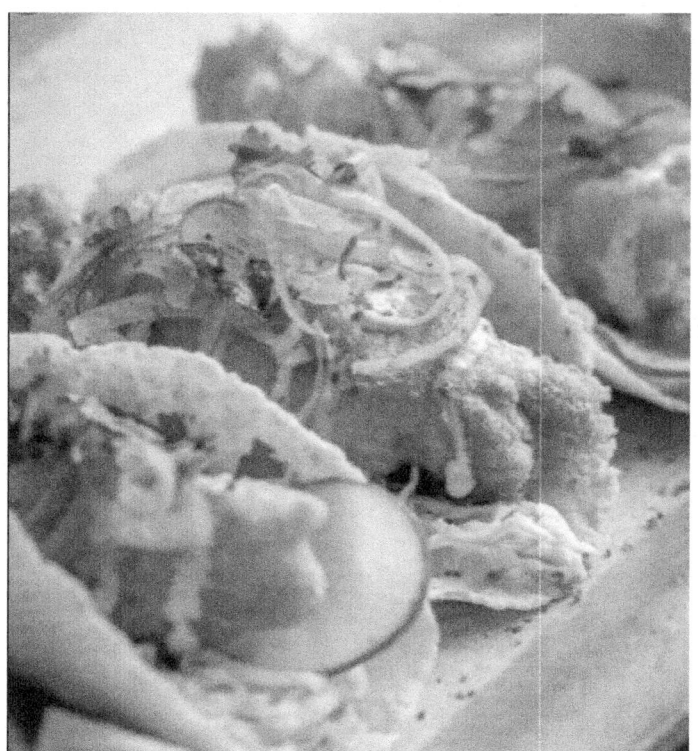

Ready in: 50mins

Yield: 8 small tacos

Ingredients

- 14 ounces silken tofu
- 1⁄2 cup plain flour
- 2 cups panko breadcrumbs
- 1⁄2 teaspoon salt
- 1⁄2 teaspoon cayenne pepper
- One teaspoon smoked paprika
- One teaspoon ground cumin
- 1⁄2 cup non-dairy milk
- 1⁄4 head cabbage, finely shredded

- vegetable oil, for frying
- One ripe avocado
- vegan mayonnaise, to serve
- Eight small tortillas

Pickled Onion

- One red onion, peeled, finely sliced
- One tablespoon sugar
- 1⁄4 cup apple cider vinegar
- One teaspoon salt

Directions

1. To extract surplus moisture, pat the tofu with a few pieces of kitchen roll. I want them to be imperfect, not cubes, because they look better! Use a knife to split the tofu into rough 1 inch pieces.
2. Place the breadcrumbs in a shallow, large cup.
3. In another large, shallow cup, place the flour, salt, smoked paprika, cayenne, and cumin and stir together.
4. Put the milk in a shallow bowl that is third deep.
5. Take the pieces of tofu and gently coat them on a baking sheet with the flour, then the milk, then the breadcrumbs.
6. Fill a deep frying pan with vegetable oil about 1/2-inch deep. Sprinkle a breadcrumb in, and if it starts to bubble and brown, the oil is hot enough. Put it over medium heat and let the oil get hot. To the oil, add chunks of breaded tofu and fry until golden underneath, then flip and cook so that it's all golden.

Remove to a baking sheet lined with a drainable kitchen roll. Repeat with the tofu that remains.

For the pickled onion:

1. Heat the vinegar, salt, and sugar from the apple cider in a small pot until steaming. Put the finely sliced red onion in a bowl or pot and pour the hot vinegar over it. To soften and turn pink, let it sit for at least 30 minutes.
2. Serve the spicy fried tofu, pickled onion, a smear of vegan mayo, some avocado, and shredded cabbage in warmed tortillas (I warm them over my stove's lit gas ring).

LUNCH

12. Mama's Supper Club Tilapia Parmesan

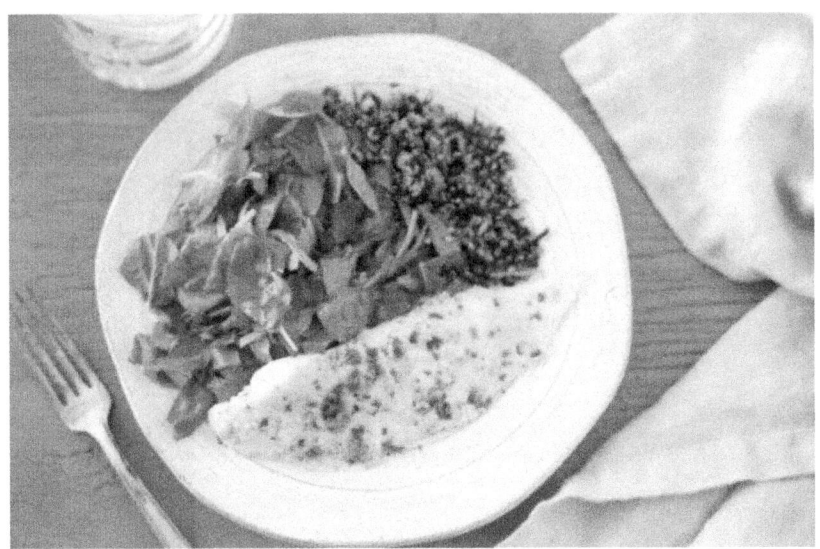

Ready in: 35mins

Serves: 4

Ingredients

- 1/2 cup grated parmesan cheese
- Two tablespoons lemon juice
- Three tablespoons mayonnaise
- Three tablespoons finely chopped green onions
- Four tablespoons butter, room temperature
- 1/4 teaspoon dried basil
- black pepper
- 1/4 teaspoon seasoning salt (I like Old Bay seasoning here)

- One dash of hot pepper sauce
- 2 lbs tilapia fillets (orange roughy, cod, or red snapper can be substituted)

Directions

1. Preheat the oven to 350°C.
2. Lay the fillets in a single layer in a buttered 13-by-9-inch baking dish or jelly roll pan.
3. Do not have fillets stacked.
4. Brush with juice on top.
5. Mix the cheese, butter, mayonnaise, onions, and seasonings in a dish.
6. Blend well with the fork.
7. In a preheated oven, bake the fish for 10 to 20 minutes or until the fish just begins to flake.
8. Spread with cheese mixture and bake for around 5 minutes, until golden brown.
9. Baking time will depend on the fish thickness that you are using.
10. Control the fish carefully so that they do not overcook.
11. Note: You can make this fish in a broiler, too.
12. Broil for 3-4 minutes or until nearly through.
13. Attach the cheese and broil for 2 to 3 minutes or until it is browned.

13. **Shredded Brussels Sprouts With Bacon And Onions**

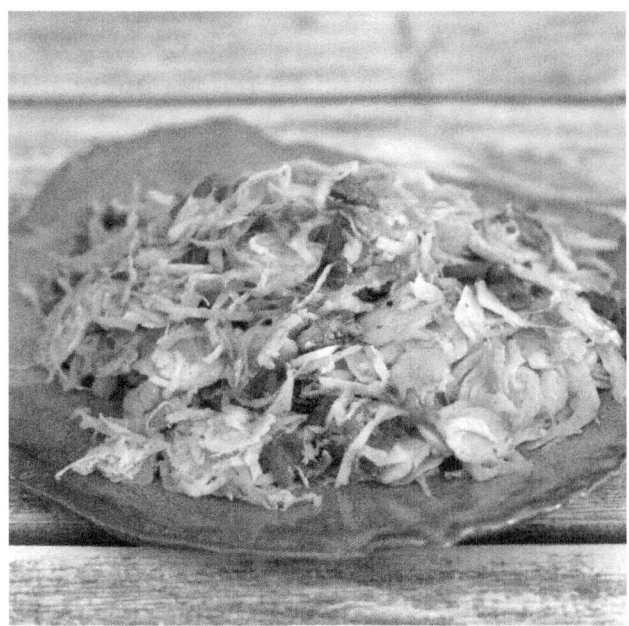

Ready in: 30mins

Serves: 6

Ingredients

- One small yellow onion, thinly sliced
- Two slices of bacon
- 3⁄4 cup water
- One teaspoon Dijon mustard
- 1⁄4 teaspoon salt (or to taste)
- One tablespoon cider vinegar
- 1 lb Brussels sprout, trimmed, halved, and very thinly sliced

Directions

1. Cook bacon in a large pan until crisp (5 to 7 minutes) over medium heat; drain on paper towels, then crumble.
2. Transfer the onion and salt to the pan's drippings and cook over medium heat until tender and browned, frequently stirring (about 3 minutes).
3. Add water and mustard, scrape any browned parts, add sprouts from Brussels and cook, stirring regularly, until tender (4 to 6 minutes).
4. Stir in the vinegar and add the crumbled bacon to the tip.

14. Roasted Broccoli W Lemon Garlic & Toasted Pine Nuts

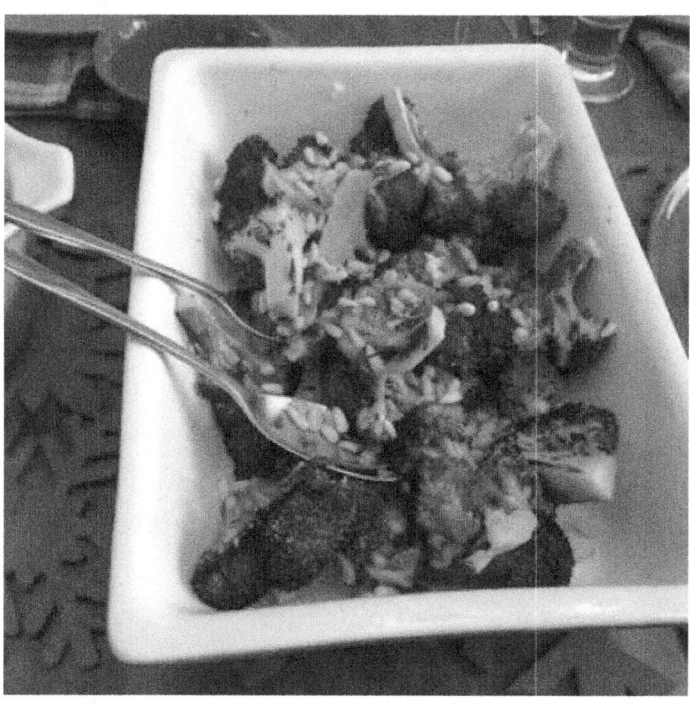

Ready in: 22mins

Serves: 4

Ingredients

- 1 lb broccoli floret
- salt & freshly ground black pepper
- Two tablespoons olive oil
- Two tablespoons unsalted butter
- 1/2 teaspoon lemon zest, grated
- One teaspoon garlic, minced
- 1 -2 tablespoon fresh lemon juice
- Two tablespoons pine nuts, toasted

Directions

1. Preheat the oven to 500°C.
2. Toss the broccoli with the oil in a wide bowl and add salt and pepper to taste.
3. On a baking sheet, arrange the florets into a single layer and roast, turning once for 12 minutes or until just tender.
4. Meanwhile, over medium heat, melt the butter in a small saucepan.
5. Apply the zest of garlic and lemon and heat for about 1 minute, stirring.
6. Let the lemon juice cool slightly and stir it in.
7. Put the broccoli in a serving bowl, pour the lemon butter over it, and toss to coat it.
8. Over the top, scatter the toasted pine nuts.

15. Cauliflower Popcorn - Roasted Cauliflower

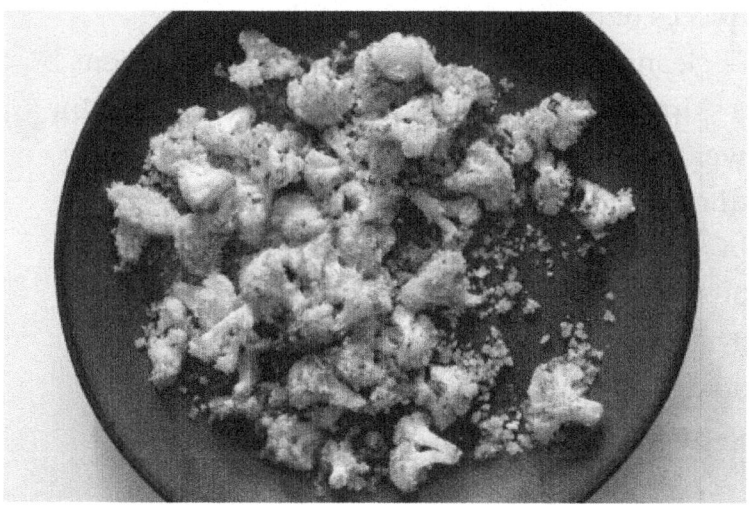

Ready in: 1hr 10mins

Serves: 4

Ingredients

- Four tablespoons olive oil
- one head cauliflower or one equal head amount of pre-cut commercially prepped cauliflower
- one teaspoon salt, to taste

Directions

1. Preheat the oven to 425°C.
2. Trim the cauliflower head, discarding the thick stems and the core; cut the florets into pieces around the ping-pong balls' size.

3. Combine the olive oil and salt in a large bowl, whisk, then add the pieces of cauliflower and toss thoroughly.
4. For quick cleaning, line a baking sheet with parchment (you can skip that, if you don't have one, then spread the cauliflower pieces on the sheet and roast for 1 hour, turning three or four times, until most of each piece turns golden brown.
5. (The browner the pieces of cauliflower turn, the more caramelization happens and the sweeter they taste).
6. Serve and drink it instantly!

16. Best Baked Potato

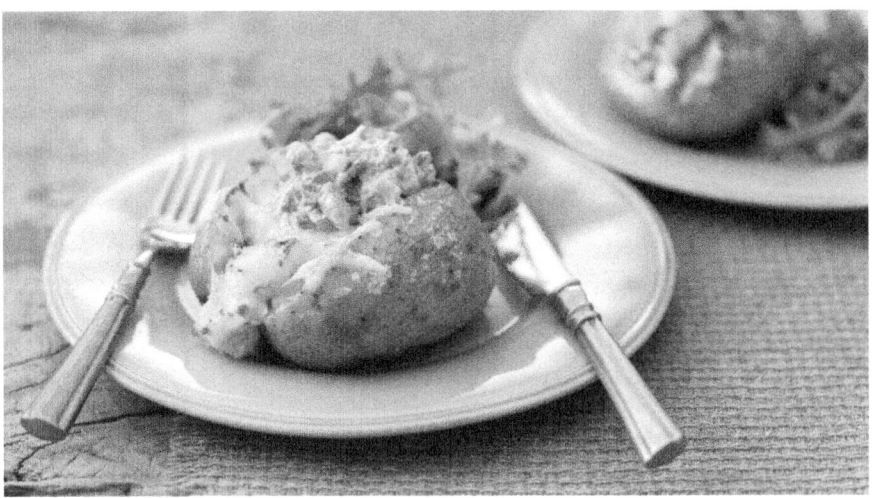

Ready in: 1hr 10mins

Serves: 1

Ingredients

- canola oil
- One large russet potato
- kosher salt

Directions

1. Heat the oven to 350 ° F and place the upper and lower thirds of the racks.
2. Thoroughly wash the potato (or potatoes) with a stiff brush and cold running water.
3. Dry, then poke 8 to 12 deep holes all over the spud using a regular fork so that moisture can escape during cooking.
4. Place it in a bowl and gently coat it with oil.
5. Sprinkle with kosher salt and put the potato in the middle of the oven directly on a rack.
6. To trap any drippings, place a baking sheet (I placed a piece of aluminum foil) on the lower rack.
7. Bake for 1 hour or until the skin feels crisp, but the flesh feels soft underneath.
8. Serve by forming a dotted line with your fork from end to end, then crack the spud open by pressing the ends towards each other.
9. It's going to pop open right.
10. But watch out, there's going to be some steam there.

NOTE: You will need to increase the cooking time by up to 15 minutes if you are cooking more than four potatoes.

17. Easy Black Bean Soup

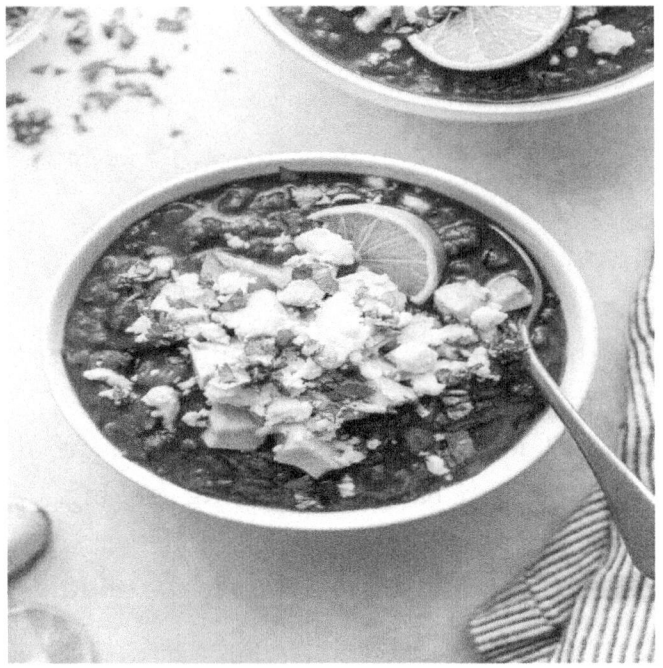

Ready in: 25mins

Serves: 4

Ingredients

- Three tablespoons olive oil
- one tablespoon ground cumin
- One medium onion, chopped
- 2 -3 cloves garlic
- two (14 1/2 ounce) cans of black beans
- salt and pepper
- two cups chicken broth or 2 cups vegetable broth

- One small red onion, chopped fine
- 1/4 cup cilantro, coarsely chopped or finely chopped (whatever you prefer)

Directions

1. In olive oil, saute the onion.
2. Add cumin when the onion becomes translucent.
3. Cook for 30 seconds, add garlic, and cook for an additional 30 to 60 seconds.
4. Add one can of vegetable broth and 2 cups of black beans.
5. Bring to a boil, sometimes stirring.
6. Turn the heat off.
7. Mix the ingredients in the pot using a hand blender, or switch them to a blender.
8. Connect the second can of beans and the mixed ingredients to the pot and bring to a simmer.
9. Serve the soup with red onion bowls and cilantro for garnishing.
10. I'm also adding a bit of cilantro to the pot.
11. It can be doubled or frozen.

18. Vegan Lentil Burgers

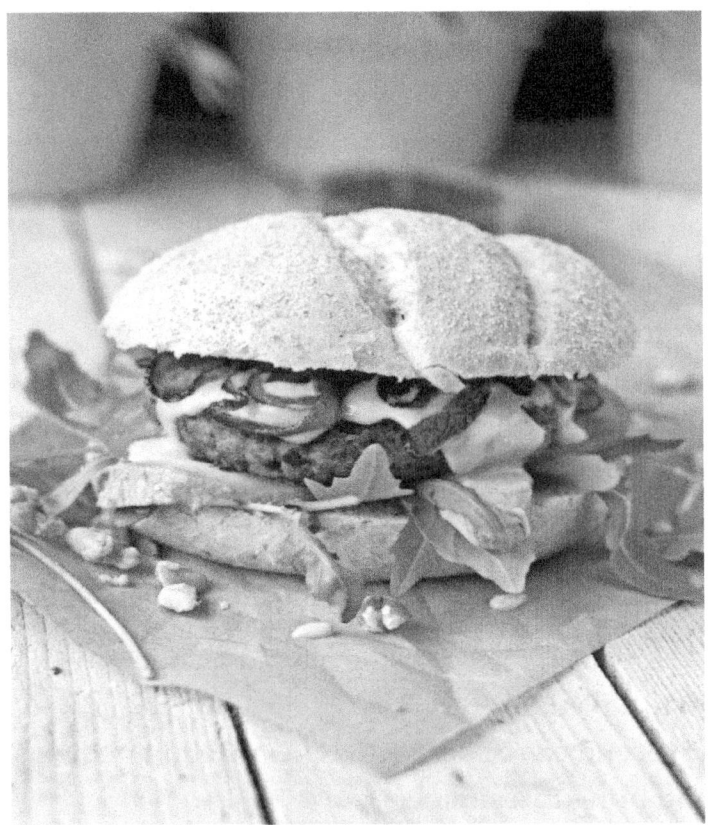

Ready in: 1hr 10mins

Yield: 8-10 burgers

Ingredients

- 2 1/2 cups water
- 1 cup dry lentils, well rinsed
- 1/2 teaspoon salt
- 1/2 medium onion, diced
- One carrot, diced
- One tablespoon olive oil
- One teaspoon pepper

- One tablespoon soy sauce
- 3⁄4 cup breadcrumbs
- 3⁄4 cup rolled oats, finely ground

Directions

1. Boil the lentils with the salt in the water for about 45 minutes. The lentils are going to be soft, and much of the water is gone.
2. It will take about 5 minutes to fry the onions and carrots in oil until tender.
3. The cooked ingredients are combined in a bowl with pepper, soy sauce, oats, and bread crumbs.
4. While the mixture is still warm, it will produce ten burgers.
5. Burgers can then be fried shallowly on each side for 1-2 minutes or baked for 15 minutes at 200C.

19. Vegan Coconut Kefir Banana Muffins

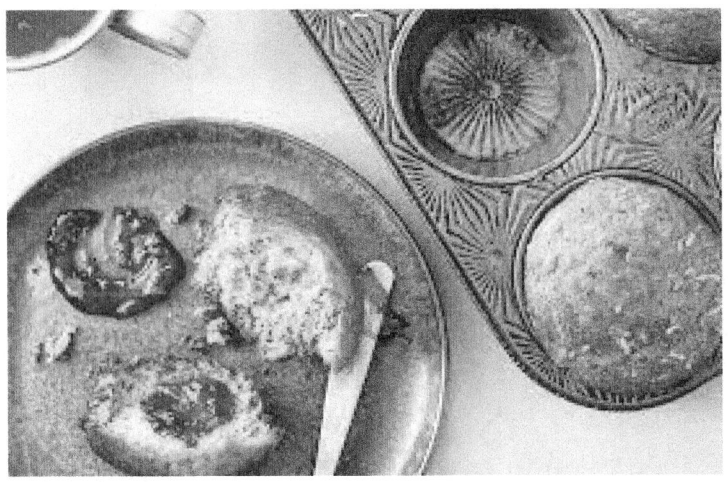

Ready in: 45mins

Serves: 12

Ingredients

- 2 cups all-purpose flour
- 1 cup unsweetened dried shredded coconut
- 1 cup granulated sugar
- Two teaspoons baking soda
- 1/2 teaspoon salt
- Two ripe bananas, mashed
- One teaspoon baking powder
- 1/4 cup cold-pressed liquid coconut oil
- 1 1/2 cups pc dairy-free kefir probiotic fermented coconut milk
- one teaspoon vanilla extract

Directions

1. Preheat the oven to 180oC (350oF). Mist 12-Count Cooking Spray Muffin Tin. Only set aside.
2. In a big bowl, whisk together the flour, sugar, coconut, baking soda, baking powder, and salt. Only set aside.
3. In a separate, large cup, whisk together the bananas, kefir, coconut oil, and vanilla. Add to the flour mixture; stir until there are no white streaks left.
4. Divide the prepared muffin tin between the wells. Cook until the tops are golden and the toothpick inserted in the centers comes out clean, about 30 minutes. Let it cool for 15 minutes in the muffin pan.
5. Chef's tip: let them cool fully on a rack to freeze muffins, then move to an airtight container or resealable freezer bag and freeze for up to a month. You may individually cover the muffins in plastic wrap or foil before placing them in the container or bag for additional protection against freezer burn. In the oven, Overnight thaw muffins or microwave straight from frozen until warmed through around 20 to 30 seconds.

20. Sauerkraut Salad

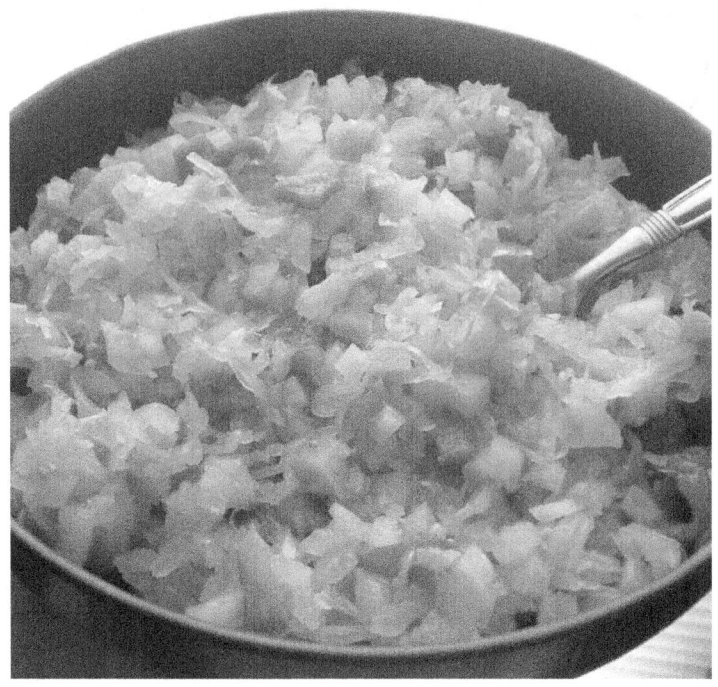

Ready in: 15mins

Serves: 6

Ingredients

- 1 cup celery, chopped fine
- 1 (1 lb) can sauerkraut, drained but not rinsed
- 1/2 cup green pepper, chopped fine
- 1/2 teaspoon salt
- Two tablespoons onions, chopped fine
- 1/2 teaspoon pepper
- 1/3 cup salad oil
- 3/4 cup sugar

- 1/3 cup cider (I use white) or 1/3 cup white vinegar (I use white)

Directions

1. Mix the sauerkraut with the chopped vegetables.
2. On low heat, heat the sugar, oil, vinegar, salt, and pepper until the sugar dissolves.
3. Refrigerate and pour over the vegetables.
4. Overnight relax.

21. Spicy Chocolate Keto Fat Bombs

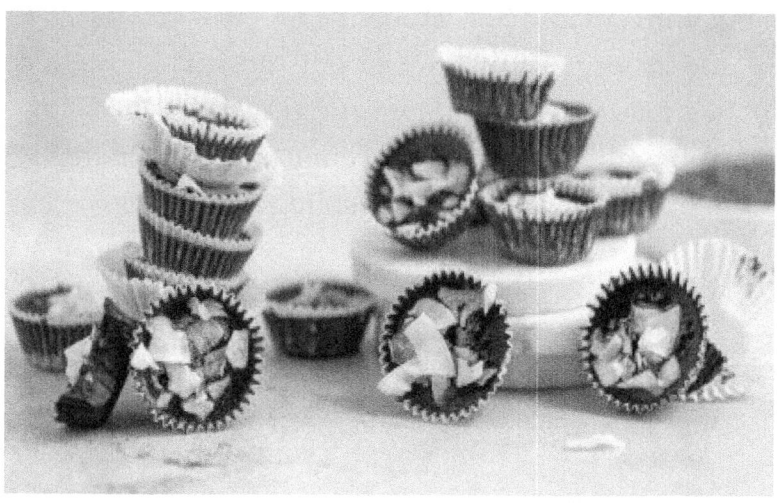

Ready in: 8mins

Serves: 24

Ingredients

- 2/3 cup coconut oil
- 1/2 cup dark cocoa
- 4 (6 g) packets stevia (or to taste)
- 2/3 cup smooth peanut butter
- One tablespoon ground cinnamon
- 1/2 cup toasted coconut flakes
- 1/4 teaspoon kosher salt
- 1/4 teaspoon cayenne (to taste)

Directions

1. In a double boiler set over a pot of simmering water, blend the coconut oil, peanut butter, and cocoa powder. Heat, whisking, until smooth and molten.
2. To mix, add stevia, cinnamon, and salt and stir.
3. Divide the mixture into a mini muffin tray made of silicone. Top with coconut and cayenne and move to the freezer for about 30 minutes, until solid.

DINNER

22. Zucchini And Eggs Recipe With Cheese

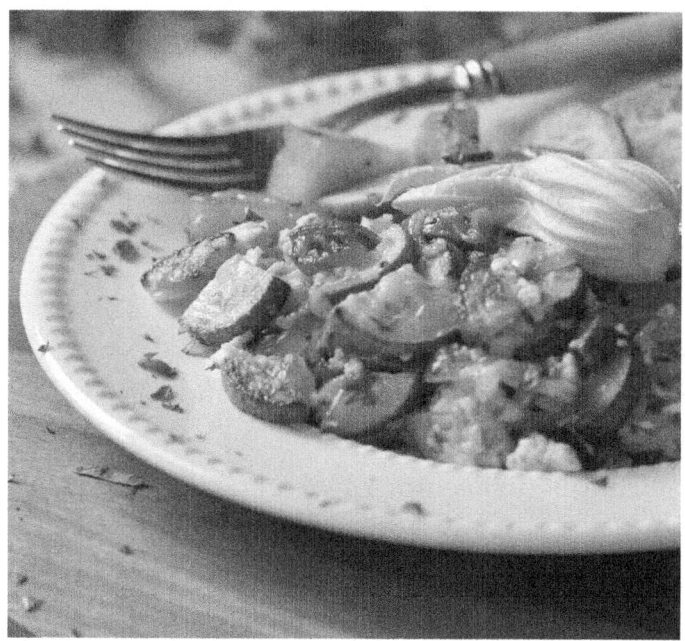

Cook Time: 16 minutes

Prep Time: 4 minutes

Total Time: 20 minutes

Servings: 1 serving

Ingredients

- One yellow onion small, sliced thinly, about 4 ounces
- One tablespoon olive oil separated
- 2-3 garlic cloves sliced in half

- One small zucchini chopped into ½-inch quarters (see note), about 6 ounces
- One egg room temperature, slightly beaten
- salt and pepper to taste
- One tablespoon water
- One tablespoon Italian parsley chopped
- 1-2 tablespoons Romano cheese grated

Instructions

1. Heat 1/2 tablespoons of olive oil over medium-high heat in a large skillet.
2. Add the onion and reduce to medium heat.
3. Cook, stirring until translucent periodically and softened for around 3-5 minutes.
4. The remaining chopped zucchini, olive oil, and garlic are added. With salt and pepper, season.
5. Saute, stirring and shaking the pan, until golden brown, over medium-high heat. It should take about 7-10 minutes for this. The zucchini needs to be baked, but it's still crisp—taste of doneness. If necessary, change the heat.
6. Meanwhile, whisk the cheese and parsley with the egg.
7. Add the egg mixture to the pan when the zucchini is cooked, and let it cook for about 30 seconds. Then stir and shake the pan until the egg is scrambled and set for 1 minute or so.
8. Taste the seasonings and change.
9. Immediately serve.
10. Garnish with chopped Italian parsley and grated cheese, if needed.

Nutrition

Serving: 1serving | Carbohydrates: 17g | Calories: 280kcal |
Protein: 10g | Fat: 20g | Saturated Fat: 4g | Sodium: 141mg |
Potassium: 529mg | Cholesterol: 169mg | Fiber: 3g | Sugar: 8g
| Iron: 2mg Vitamin A: 811IU | Vitamin C: 36mg | Calcium:
133mg |

23. Egg Scramble With Sweet Potatoes

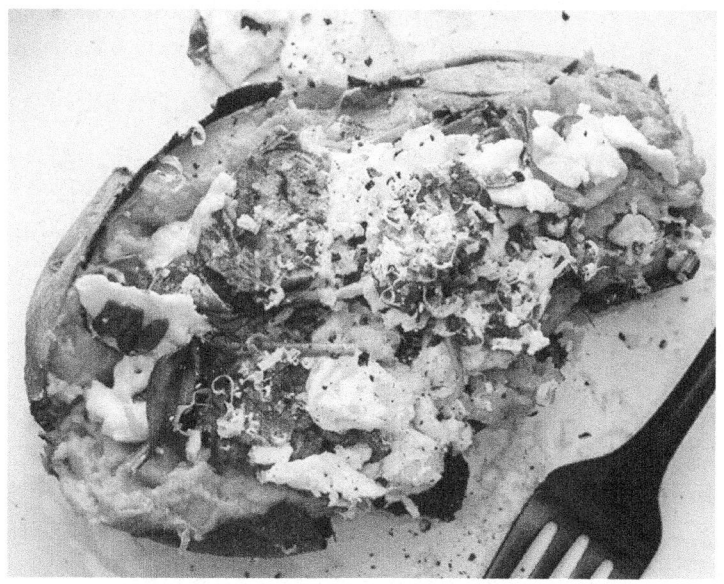

Ingredients:

- ½ cup chopped onion
- 1 (8-oz) sweet potato, diced
- 2 tsp chopped rosemary
- Salt
- Four large eggs
- Four large egg whites

- Pepper
- 2 tbsp chopped chive

Directions:

1. Preheat the heater to 425 degrees F. Toss the sweet potato, onion, rosemary, salt, and pepper on a baking dish. Spray with cooking spray and roast for about 20 minutes, until tender.
2. Meanwhile, whisk the eggs, egg whites, and a pinch of salt and pepper together in a medium cup. Spritz a cooking spray skillet and scramble the eggs over medium heat for around 5 minutes.
3. Sprinkle and serve with the spuds with chopped chives.
4. 571 calories per serving, 44 g of protein, 52 g of carbohydrates (9 g of fibre), 20 g of fat

24. Spicy Spanish Tomato Baked Eggs

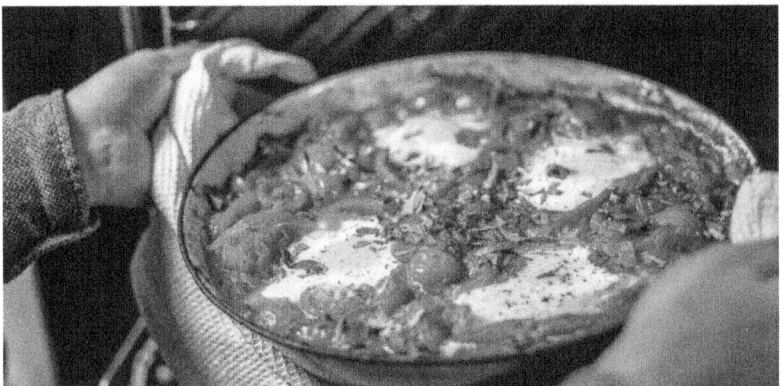

Ingredients

- One tbsp olive oil
- One red pepper, deseeded and cut into strips
- Two red onions, peeled and cut into half-moons
- One clove garlic, peeled and sliced
- 1 tsp paprika
- Four medium eggs
- 250g cherry tomatoes, halved or one tin peeled plum tomatoes
- Two tbsp chopped flat-leaf parsley (optional)

Directions

1. Preheat the oven to 180 ° C/Gas 6 200 ° C/fan
2. Heat the oil in a large, deep, ovenproof frying pan,
3. Add the onions, garlic, and pepper. Season with freshly ground black pepper and cook until soft or for 10 minutes.
4. Add the tomatoes and paprika and cook gently for an additional 5 minutes.
5. In the mixture, make four little wells and crack an egg into each. Season, cover, and place in the oven with black pepper.
6. Cook until the eggs are set - this should take 5-8 minutes or so. If used, sprinkle over the parsley.

25. Vegetable Meatloaf With Balsamic Glaze

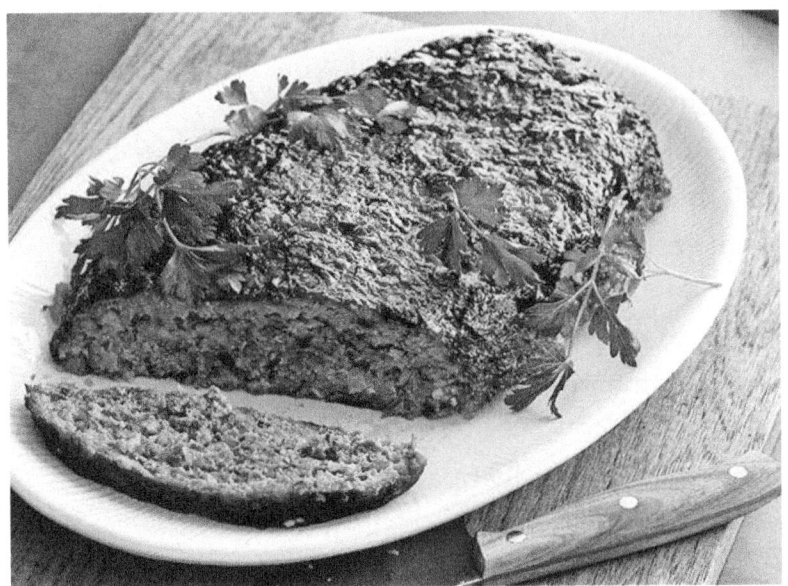

Ingredients

- Two tablespoons extra-virgin olive oil
- One small zucchini, finely diced
- One large egg, lightly beaten
- One red bell pepper, finely diced
- One yellow bell pepper, finely diced
- Five cloves garlic smashed to a paste with coarse salt
- Kosher salt and freshly ground pepper
- 1/4 cup chopped fresh parsley
- 1/2 cup Parmesan cheese or freshly grated Romano
- 1 1/2 pounds ground turkey (90% lean)
- 1 cup panko (coarse Japanese breadcrumbs)
- One tablespoon finely chopped fresh thyme
- 1/4 cup plus two tablespoons balsamic vinegar
- 3/4 cup ketchup

Directions

1. The oven should be preheated to 425 degrees. Over high pressure, heat the oil in a large saute pan. Add the zucchini, garlic paste, bell peppers, and 1/4 teaspoon of red pepper flakes. Season with pepper and salt and cook for about 5 minutes, until the vegetables are almost tender. Set to cool aside.
2. In a large cup, whisk in the egg and fresh herbs. Add turkey, panko, grated cheese, 1/2 cup of ketchup, two tablespoons of cooled vegetables, and balsamic vinegar; blend until just mixed.
3. Press the mixture into a 9-by-5-inch loaf pan gently. In a small bowl, whisk the remaining 1/4 cup balsamic vinegar and1/4 cup ketchup, 1/4 teaspoon red pepper flakes; brush the blend over the whole loaf. For 1 to 1 1/4 hours, bake. Until slicing, let it rest for 10 minutes.

26. Easy Bbq Chicken Tostadas

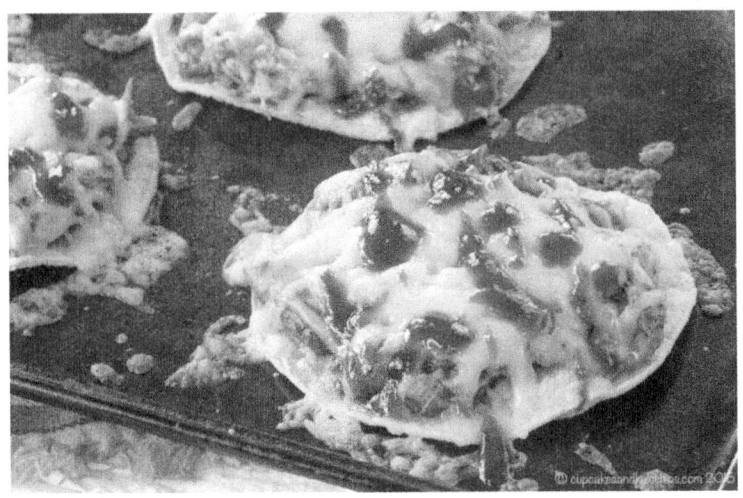

Prep Time10 mins

Total Time18 mins

Cook Time8 mins

Servings: 4

Ingredients

- Three cups cooked and shredded chicken
- One 1/2 cups of your favorite barbecue sauce, divided
- Eight tostada shells or eight corn tortillas brushed lightly with olive oil and baked for 3-5 minutes per side, until crispy
- Three green onions, very thinly sliced (optional)
- Two cups shredded cheese (Mary uses mozzarella in the cookbook, but I have also used cheddar, Monterey Jack, or a blend)

Instructions

1. Preheat to 350°F in your oven. Spread out two rimmed baking sheets with the tostada shells (or baked tortillas).
2. In a small bowl, mix the chicken and 1 cup barbecue sauce, and swirl to coat.
3. Divide the chicken between the shells of the tostada and top with the cheese (approximately 1⁄4 cup each).
4. Bake, only until the cheese is melted, for 6 to 8 minutes.
5. Remove and drizzle with the remaining 1⁄2 cup of barbecue sauce from the oven. If needed, sprinkle it with green onions.

Nutrition

Serving: 2tostadas | Vitamin A: 825IU | Calories: 693kcal | Carbohydrates: 66g | Protein: 31g | Fat: 33g | Saturated Fat: 13g | Sodium: 1730mg | Potassium: 554mg | Fiber: 3g | Sugar: 36g | Vitamin C: 3.7mg | Calcium: 359mg | Cholesterol: 107mg | Iron: 2.3mg

27. Buffalo Chicken Sandwich With Blue Cheese Slaw

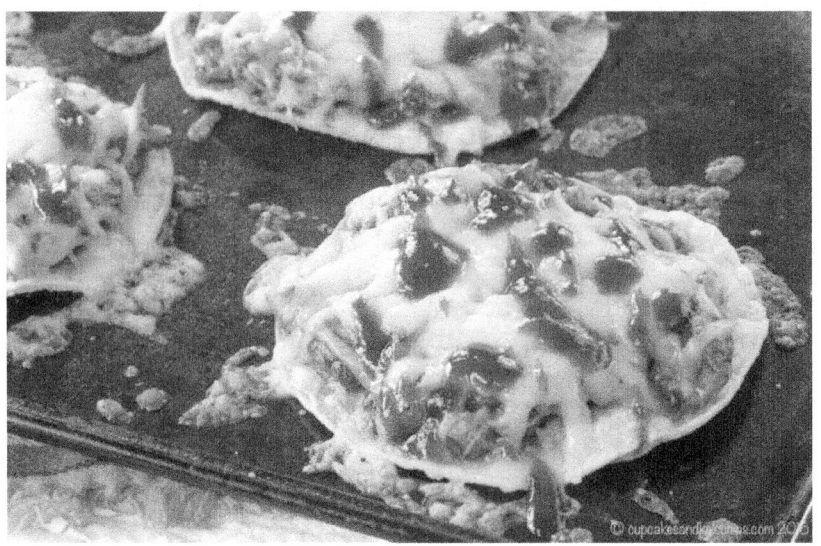

Ingredients

Blue Cheese Slaw:

- 1/4 cup mayonnaise
- One tablespoon minced garlic
- 1/4 cup crumbled blue cheese
- Two tablespoons Worcestershire sauce
- 1 (10-ounce) package coleslaw mix
- Kosher salt
- One lemon, juiced
- Freshly cracked black pepper
- Canola oil, to fry

Buffalo Chicken:

- 1/2 cup buffalo hot sauce, store-bought
- Two tablespoons smoked paprika, plus more for seasoning
- 4 (6-ounce) boneless, skinless chicken cutlets

- One tablespoon kosher salt, plus more for seasoning
- One cup self-rising flour
- 1 1/4 cups buttermilk
- Two tablespoons hot sauce
- One egg
- One tablespoon cracked black pepper, plus more for seasoning
- Four soft-club rolls, split and toasted

Directions

1. Mix the mayonnaise, crumbled blue cheese, garlic, Worcestershire sauce, and lemon juice in a medium-sized bowl until well mixed. Attach the mix of coleslaw and toss well. With salt and pepper, season and set aside.
2. Heat enough canola oil in a deep-fryer or heavy-bottomed pot to get halfway up the sides of the pot to 350 degrees F.
3. In a shallow dish, add buffalo sauce and set aside. To taste, season the chicken with smoked paprika and salt and pepper. In a shallow dish, place the flour, two tablespoons of paprika, one tablespoon of salt, and one tablespoon of pepper. Put the egg, buttermilk, and hot sauce together in another shallow dish and whisk together. Dredge each piece of chicken, shake off any excess in the buttermilk mixture, and then dredge it into the flour mixture. Fry until the chicken is cooked for around 4 to 6 minutes. On an instant-read thermometer, the internal temperature registers 165 degrees F. In the buffalo sauce, dip the finished chicken and place it on the club rolls. Top the

chicken and shape a sandwich with a liberal quantity of slaw.

28. Italian Chicken

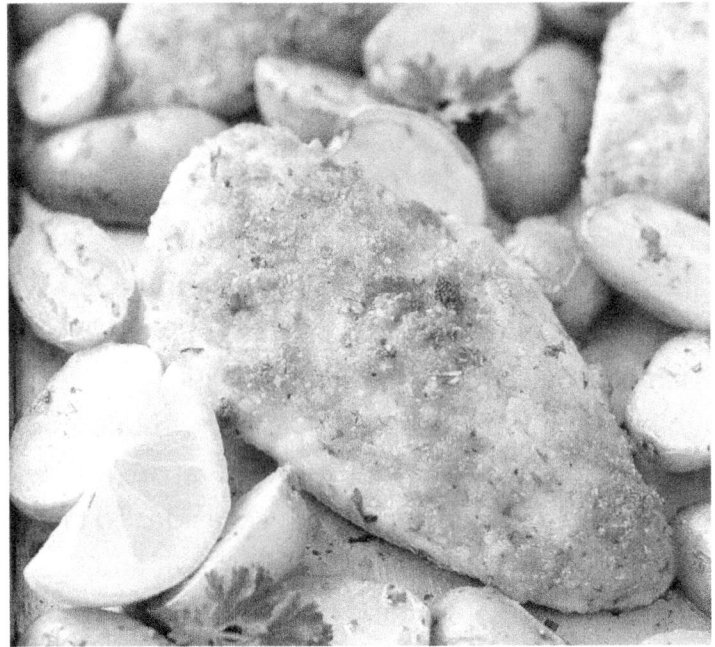

Cook Time30 minutes

Prep Time10 minutes

Total Time40 minutes

Ingredients

- Four boneless skinless chicken breasts
- 1/2 cup breadcrumbs

- 1/2 cup grated parmesan cheese
- 1/2 teaspoon minced garlic
- salt and pepper to taste
- Four tablespoons butter melted
- One teaspoon Italian seasoning
- 1 pound small potatoes halved or quartered
- cooking spray
- Two tablespoons chopped parsley
- lemon wedges optional garnish

Directions

1. To 400 degrees, preheat the oven. Using cooking spray to cover a sheet pan.
2. Mix the parmesan cheese, breadcrumbs, garlic, Italian seasoning, salt, and pepper in a small cup.
3. In the melted butter, dip the top of each chicken breast, then press the chicken's top into the breadcrumb mixture to coat it.
4. On the prepared sheet pan, put the chicken breasts.
5. About the chicken, scatter the potatoes. Drizzle over the potatoes and chicken with the remaining butter. With salt and pepper, season the potatoes.
6. Bake for 25-30 minutes or until the chicken is completely cooked and the potatoes are tender. Depending on the thickness of your chicken, the cooking time can vary.
7. Sprinkle and serve with parsley. If needed, garnish with lemon wedges.

Nutrition

Carbohydrates: 10g | Calories: 336kcal | Protein: 30g | Fat: 18g | Saturated Fat: 10g | Cholesterol: 113mg | Vitamin A: 490IU | Potassium: 460mg | Vitamin C: 1.3mg | Sodium: 520mg | Calcium: 172mg | Iron: 1.2mg

29. Oriental Turkey Burgers

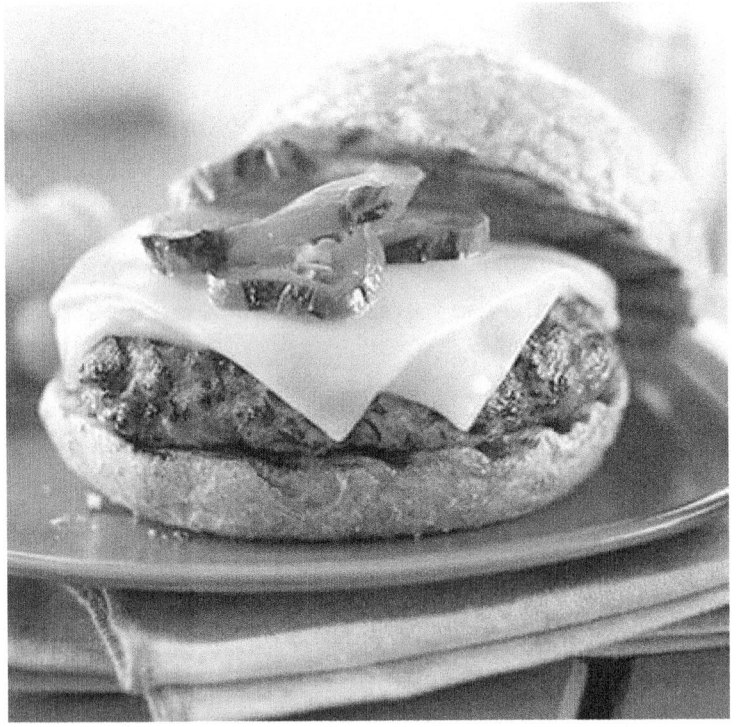

Ingredients

SLAW

- 2 cups coleslaw mix

- One tablespoon seasoned rice vinegar
- Three tablespoons chopped fresh cilantro
- One teaspoon vegetable oil

BURGER

- Two tablespoons Butter
- Two jalapeño chile peppers, seeded, finely chopped
- 1/3 cup chopped green onions
- 1 1/4 pounds lean ground turkey
- One tablespoon hoisin sauce
- One tablespoon soy sauce
- 1/4 cup dry bread crumbs
- One tablespoon butter, melted
- Hoisin sauce, if desired
- 5 (10-inch) tortillas

Directions

1. heat the gas grill until the coals are ash white on a medium or charcoal grill.
2. In a tub, mix all the slaw ingredients; mix well. Cover; leave to cool before serving time.
3. Melt two tablespoons of butter until sizzling in a 10-inch skillet; add the onion and chili peppers. Cook for approximately 1-2 minutes or until tender. Cool.
4. In a cup, combine the onion mix, turkey, bread crumbs, one tablespoon of hoisin sauce, and soy sauce; mix gently. Shape into four patties (3/4 inches thick).
5. Set the patties on the grill—a molten butter brush. Grill, rotating once, 20-30 minutes or until the inner temperature

reaches a minimum of 165 °f and the middle of the meat is no longer pink.

6. Wrap the aluminum foil tortillas. Place them away from direct heat on the grill. Move tortillas often when grilling burgers.

7. Place half of each warm tortilla with the burgers. Top with slaw; drizzle, if necessary, with hoisin sauce. Fold your tortilla over your burger.

30. Easy Shepherd's Pie Recipe

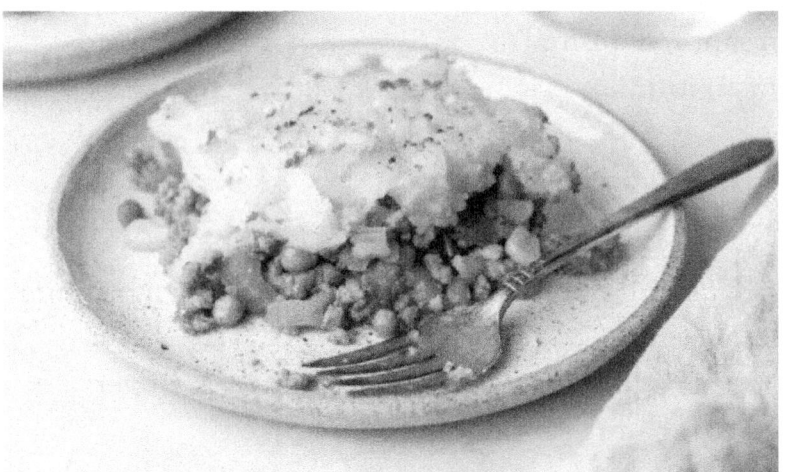

Cook time: 50 minutes

Prep time: 15 minutes

Ingredients

- 8 Tablespoons (1 stick) butter
- 1 1/2 to 2 pounds potatoes (about three large potatoes), peeled and quartered
- One medium onion, chopped (about 1 1/2 cups)
- 1 1/2 lbs ground round beef
- 1-2 cups vegetables—diced carrots, corn, peas
- 1/2 cup beef broth
- Salt, pepper, other seasonings of choice
- One teaspoon Worcestershire sauce

Instructions

1. Boil the potatoes: Place the peeled and quartered potatoes in a medium-sized bath. Cover for at least an inch with cold water. There is a teaspoon of salt added. Bring to a boil, simmer, and cook, then reduce to a simmer until tender (about 20 minutes).

2. Sauté vegetables: Melt four tablespoons of butter over medium heat in a large saucepan while frying the potatoes. Attach the chopped onions and cook them until tender for approximately 6 to 10 minutes.

Add them if you have vegetables, according to their cooking time. Carrots should be baked with onions, as they take as long to cook as onions.

Add them at the end of the onion cooking process or after the meat starts to cook if peas or corn are included, as they take very little time to cook.

3. Add the ground beef and then the Worcestershire sauce and the broth: add the onions and vegetables to the ground beef pan. Cook until there's no pinker. With salt and pepper, season.

Add the beef broth and Worcestershire sauce. Simmer the broth and reduce the heat to a low level. To prevent the meat from drying out, cook uncovered for 10 minutes, adding more beef broth if necessary.

4. Mash the cooked potatoes: When the potatoes are cooked, remove them from the pot and put them in a bowl with the remaining four Teaspoons of butter (a fork will easily pierce). With a fork or potato masher, mash and season to taste with salt and pepper.

5. Arrange the meat mixture in a casserole dish with the mashed potatoes: Preheat the oven to 400 °F. In a bread baking dish, spread the beef, onions, and vegetables (if used) in an even layer (9x1 casserole).

On top of the ground beef, spread the mashed potatoes over the top. Using a fork to rough up the mashed potatoes' surface so that there are peaks that get well browned. You can also use a fork to render the mashed potatoes with innovative designs.

6. Bake in the oven: Put in the oven at 400°F and cook for about 30 minutes until browned and bubbling. To help the surface of the mashed potatoes brown, broil for the last few minutes if necessary.

(When broiling using Pyrex or glass dishes, it is understood that they break under the broiler's high heat. Whether you are using a ceramic or metal casserole dish, it is not a concern.)

Chapter 23: 16/8 INTERMITTENT FASTING PLAN FOR 21 DAYS

WEEK 1

DAY 1

8: 00am: Warm Lemon Honey Water

11:00 am - Breakfast: ½ Chees/Bagel/Egg/Coconut Cream/Coffee

3:00 pm - Snack: Kind Bar

5:00 pm - Diner: Green Beans with Sauteed Chicken Breast

Brown Rice

7:00 pm – Fasting

DAY 2

8:00 am: Warm Lemon Honey Water

11:00 am - BREAKFAST: Coconut Creamer/Greek Yogurt/Coffee

3:00 pm - SNACK: Apple Slices

5:00 pm - DINNER: Steamed Broccoli, Grilled Salmon, Brown Rice

7:00 pm - Fasting

DAY 3

8:00 am: Warm Lemon Honey Water

11:00 am - BREAKFAST: Almond Butter/Oatmeal

Coffee/Coconut Creamer

3:00 pm - SNACK: Nuts

5:00 pm - DINNER: Tomatoes/Sauteed Egg

Brown Rice

7:00 pm: Fasting

DAY 4

8:00 am – Warm Lemon Honey Water

11:00 am – BREAKFAST: Coconut Creamer/Coffee

Avocado Toast/Egg

3:00 pm – SNACK: Banana/Strawberry Smoothie

5:00 pm – DINNER: Steamed Broccoli

Teriyaki Chicken

Brown Rice

7:00 pm – Fasting

DAY 5

8:00 am – Warm Lemon Honey Water

11:00 am – BREAKFAST: Triple Berry Smoothies

Coconut Creamer/Coffee

3:00 pm – SNACK: Nuts

5:00 pm – DINNER: Cauliflower Rice with Sauteed Chicken and Mushroom

7:00 pm- Fasting

DAY 6

8:00 am – Warm Lemon Honey Water

11:00 am – BREAKFAST: Whole Wheat Pancake

Coconut Creamer/Coffee

3:00 pm – SNACK: Blueberries

5:00 pm – DINNER: Dine Out

7:00 pm – Fasting

DAY 7

8:00 am – Warm Lemon Honey Water

9:00 am – Coconut Milk with Coffee

11:00 am – Breakfast Skip

3:00 ppm – SNACK: Nuts

5:00 pm - DINNER: Ground Pork and Spinach with Soba Noodle

7:00 pm: Fasting

WEEK 2

DAY 8

8:00 am: Lemon water

8:30 am: Skip breakfast

12:00 pm: Avocado chicken salad

3:00 pm: Nuts

7:00 pm: Macadamia basil pesto pasta

8:00 pm: Begin fasting

DAY 9

8:00 am: Black coffee

8:30 am: Skip breakfast

12:00 pm: Vegan chickpea salad

3:00 pm: Fruit of your choice

7:00 pm: Mexican tempeh

8:00 pm: Begin fasting

DAY 10

8:00 am: Black coffee

8:30 am: Skip breakfast

12:00 pm: Tuna avocado salad wrap

3:00 pm: Hummus & raw veggie sticks

7:00 pm: Asian fried noodles

8:00 pm: Begin fasting

DAY 11

8:00 am: Apple cider vinegar drink

8:30 am: Skip breakfast

12:00 pm: Broccoli tofu salad

3:00 pm: Dark chocolate

7:00 pm: Salmon kale salad

8:00 pm: Begin fasting

DAY 12

8:00 am: Lemon water

8:30 am: Skip breakfast

12:00 pm: Turkey chili

3:00 pm: Organic edamamae

7:00 pm: Grilled chicken salad

8:00 pm: Begin fasting

DAY 13

8:00 am: Lemon water

8:30 am: Skip breakfast

12:00 pm: Grilled salmon

3:00 pm: Dark chocolate bark

7:00 pm: Chicken tortilla soup

8:00 pm: Begin fasting

DAY 14

8: 00 am: Black coffee

8:30 am: Skip breakfast

12:00 pm: Sprouts, chicken, quinoa Buddah bowl

3:00 pm: Greek yogurt

7:00 pm: Teriyaki chicken with cauliflower rice

8:00 pm: Begin fasting

WEEK 3

DAY 15

8:00 am: Lemon water

8:30 am: Skip breakfast

12:00 pm: Grilled salmon

3:00 pm: Dark chocolate bark

7:00 pm: Chicken tortilla soup

8:00 pm: Begin fasting

DAY 16

8:00 am: Black coffee

8:30 am: Skip

12:00 pm: Mexican chicken tortilla Soup

3:00 pm: Handful of nuts

7:00 pm: Chicken avocado mixed green salad

8:00 pm: Begin fasting

Day 17

8:00 am: Lemon water

8:30 am: Skip

12:00 pm: Chocolate peanut butter shake

3:00 pm: Roll fried zuchinni + smoke salmon

7:00 pm: Beef Stroganoff over Cauliflower mash

8:00 pm: Begin fasting

Day 18

8:00 am: Apple cider vinegar drink

8:30 am: Skip

12:00 pm: Tuna Avocado salad wrap

3:00 pm: Hummus + raw vegie sticks

7:00 pm: Asian fried "noodles"

8:00 pm: Begin fasting

Day 19

8:00 am: Lemon water

8:30 am: Skip

12:00 pm: Egg salad

3:00 pm: Piece of dark chocolate

7:00pm: Salmon kale salad

8:00 pm: Begin fasting

Day 20

8:00 am: Black coffee

8:30 am: Skip

12:00 pm: Turkey chili

3:00 pm: Organic Edamame

7:00 pm: Grilled chicken salad

8:00 pm: Begibn fasting

Day 21

8:00 am: Apple cider vinegar drink

12:00 pm: Grilled salmon salad

3:00 pm: Dark chocolate bark

7:00 pm: Chicken tortilla soup

8:00 pm: Begin fasting

CONCLUSION

In conclusion, IF is a diet that is simple and safe and makes dieting enjoyable. Although it contradicts many of today's ideas and views, there is science behind it. You'd think that with all of these new ideas and diets, the world would be getting more fit, rather than the obesity rate reaching an all-time high. Studies and science show Intermittent Fasting works, and if the Romans, the peak of fitness, used it to stay fit, why shouldn't we.

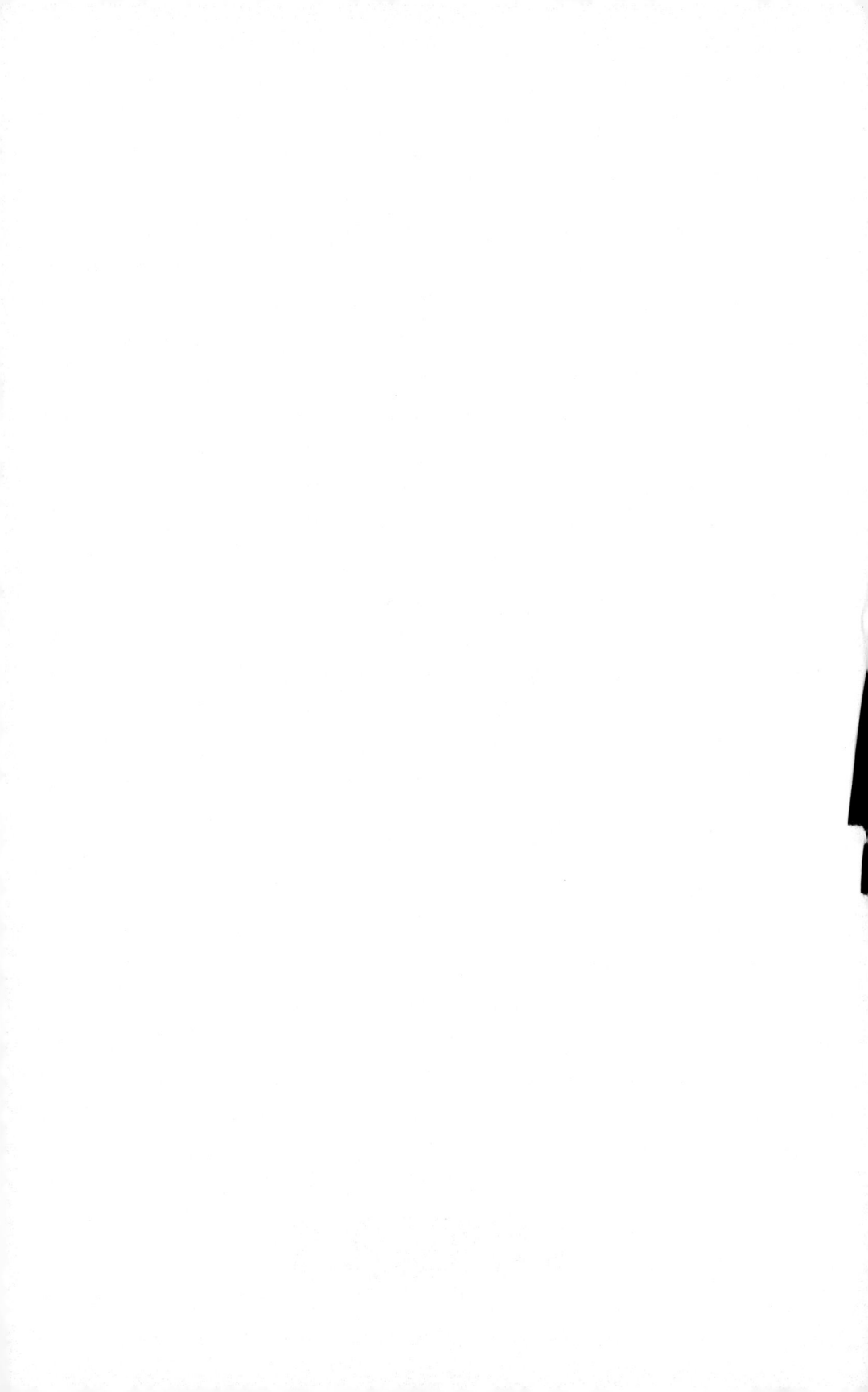

Made in the USA
Monee, IL
14 August 2022

11627134R00144